FOUNDATIONS
OF
CONDITIONING

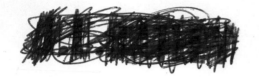

FOUNDATIONS OF CONDITIONING

HAROLD B. FALLS
Southwest Missouri State College

EARL L. WALLIS
San Fernando Valley California State College

GENE A. LOGAN
University of Southern California

ACADEMIC PRESS
New York and London

Text and cover design by Ben Kann

Copyright © 1970 by Academic Press, Inc.
All rights reserved
No part of this book may be reproduced in any form, by
photostat, microfilm, retrieval system, or any other means,
without written permission from the publishers.

ACADEMIC PRESS, INC.
111 Fifth Avenue, New York, N.Y. 10003

United Kingdom Edition published by
ACADEMIC PRESS, INC. (LONDON) LTD.
Berkeley Square House, London W1X 6BA

Library of Congress Catalog Card Number: 77–117082

Printed in the United States of America

Contents

Preface

Never before have we as clearly understood the need for exercise to promote and maintain human well-being and personal effectiveness. This need has been convincingly shown through research in medicine, physiology, and other related fields. As a result of these scientific investigations our understanding of physical conditioning has advanced significantly in recent years. This persuasive new knowledge has led us to reappraise and often reshape the guiding principles upon which a scientific conditioning program rests.

Educated people realize that physical activity is essential for optimal health. There is continuing widespread concern throughout society over the low level of fitness. Yet little is done about it. Sedentary college students enter sedentary professional lives in which they have busy schedules and often lack the desire to engage in activity, although they think they should. Frequently they do not know what constitutes an effective exercise program. They experiment with exercise fads and diet fads without realizing that there is no quick and easy way to guarantee fitness. There are, however, efficient ways to employ exercise stresses which will result in the desired adaptations.

It is the intent of this book to present authoritative information as a logical basis for the development and maintenance of physical fitness. The why as well as the how is presented. Too often people have been exercised rather than educated. If there is a rational basis for it, regular activity is more likely to be practiced, to become a part of one's style of life and value system. It is for this reason that this book emphasizes understanding of the effect of activity on fitness. The ideas presented are well documented and substantiated by research.

This book deals primarily with information about strength, flexibility, and endurance which are the basic elements of physical fitness. The specific exercises to develop these characteristics are pictured and described in detail. Also described are the modifications the body makes to the stress of exercise resulting in such adaptations as the general improvement in metabolic processes, increased working capacity, body weight control, and the improvement of cardiovascular health.

This book is designed primarily for university and college students in such typical courses as Foundations of Physical Activity, Physical Fitness, Body Conditioning, etc., but others may find it useful and informative. This is a marked departure from the traditions of books of this type in that emphasis Is placed on knowledge and understanding as well as performing. It is believed that this approach is more likely to develop an appreciation of the need for exercise. With rationality as motivation, activity is more likely to become an important part of the value structure of daily living.

The authors would like to thank Bill H. Armstrong of Southwest Missouri State College for his illustrations of the exercise techniques.

FOUNDATIONS
OF
CONDITIONING

ONE/
Adaptations
to Exercise
Stresses

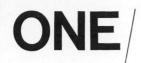

ONE/

I. PHYSIOLOGICAL ADAPTATION TO EXERCISE DEMANDS

Affluent contemporary Man has developed a technological society in which his biological organism is seldom required to perform vigorously to provide for his daily requirements. He is born with a potentiality that he need not use. In less than a century scientific innovation, the development of automation, computers, and an endless variety of laborsaving devices, has produced an environment which is actually alien, in many ways, to the organism which has evolved over millions of years. During the evolutionary process physiological adaptations kept pace with environmental changes. Man is equipped with a body capable of and requiring vigorous activity, but the necessity for its use has diminished.

The drastic change in necessary activity occurring in a short period of time has provided little opportunity for further organismic adaptations. Man has had no "natural" opportunity to adapt to the present-day mode of existence. Instead, as a thinking animal he has discovered that he must provide for his physical activity requirements through what may be considered artificial means. Mounting evidence indicates that many of Man's current illness problems are what Kraus and Raab (1961) call *hypokinetic diseases* (diseases produced by lack of exercise). Bortz (1960) has pointed out that many patients seek treatment by physicians for conditions which could be avoided by a moderate effort to keep fit. He, among others, has presented persuasive evidence that inactivity leads to deterioration. Living is a dynamic phenomenon with the tissues continually changing.

Although evolutionary adjustments to environment are made slowly, the body has a remarkable ability to make adaptations as stresses are imposed upon it. A gradual progressive adaptation to the stress of muscular work results in an increased ability to perform subsequent muscular activity. However, such adaptation is reversible: the less one does, the less one is capable of doing. Yet, barring disease other than the hypokinetic type, after resumption of exercise the body may adapt to imposed stresses and improve its capacity to function, regardless of the duration of inactivity. An adaptation continuum is illustrated (Figure 1.1) suggesting the positive and negative effects of exercise that vary in relation to the amount and intensity of imposed demands.

A. Imposed Demands

With available time for leisure increasing rapidly and sedentary existence becoming the mode of living, the adaptations necessary for optimum physiological functioning of the organism can be made for most

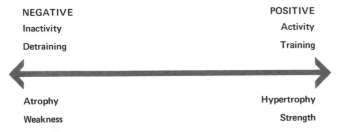

NEGATIVE   POSITIVE

Inactivity   Activity

Detraining   Training

Atrophy   Hypertrophy

Weakness   Strength

FIGURE 1.1
Adaptation Continuum.
Negative results (left)
of inactivity and detraining
include atrophy of muscles
and weakness. Activity
and training (right) result
in muscle hypertrophy and
strength.

persons only by supplementary physical activity. Man must seek ways to develop and maintain his condition. A guiding principle has been advanced for the achievement of physical fitness. It provides for maximum effect with a minimum of effort and time consumption. This concept has been called the *SAID* principle (Wallis and Logan, 1964). The principle is derived from a coined word representing the first letter in the expression "Specific Adaptation to *Imposed Demands*." This principle has been applied in the design of the exercise programs presented in this book. The application of the SAID principle leads to a most effective and efficient application of exercise.

B. Physical Fitness Elements

The physical fitness elements—strength, endurance, and flexibility—are biological bodily adjustments which are developed gradually according to the stress applied. These adjustments are reversible. As a result of disuse the individual becomes less strong, less flexible, and has less endurance. Exercise, if sufficiently intense, increases the capacity to perform more exercise. It is the only activity which provides the means to improved fitness and body conformation. Without exercise, muscles become lax and flabby, no longer holding the body in shape and no longer having the capacity to contract forcefully or the ability to sustain effort for a period of time. The axiom that form tends to follow function applies to the human body.

Continued demands must be placed upon the body in order that the elements of physical fitness be maintained at a high level. Maintenance actually results from application of small doses of stress. This prevents the reversal of the state of fitness resulting from disuse of the body.

Although the development of the physical fitness elements of strength, endurance, and flexibility are presented in later chapters, certain values of these factors might well be mentioned here. Strength, the ability to exert muscular force, is of value in several ways. It allows the individual to perform better the skills required for daily living; it contributes greatly to the effective performance of sports skills. Obviously, the amount of strength required depends upon the activity or sport in question. Adequate strength is required to maintain comfortable, balanced postures. Although Wells (1966) points out that stronger muscles do not necessarily assure better posture, good posture requires at least normal muscular strength. Endurance, the ability to sustain prolonged activity, is essential to provide for movement efficiency. As endurance is developed the energy required to perform a given amount of work is decreased and the onset of fatigue is delayed. And finally, adequate flexibility, the range of motion of bodily parts, is necessary for efficient movement. Too little or too much flexibility may be detrimental. There appears to be an optimum level of flexibility depending upon the type of activity in which an individual participates. Normal flexibility development for the person whose living is generally sedentary involves sufficient activity to compensate for shortening adaptations made in connective tissue due to inactivity.

C. Exercise Tolerance

The capacity and tolerance for exercise varies with physical condition and age of the individual. Regardless of the age of the individual, exercise can be of benefit if it is judiciously applied. The level of performance must always be within the person's capacity. Too often, attempting exercises which are beyond one's tolerance is the cause of muscular strain. However, it should be noted that no scientific evidence is available indicating harmful effects from regular exercise in the healthy person. The importance of periodic physical examinations by a physician to chart the health status of the individual cannot be stressed too strongly.

II. SCIENTIFIC BASES FOR EXERCISE

Today's science of conditioning is *not* the same science of 50, 25, or even 10 years ago. As in all rapidly developing fields of knowledge we must con-

tinually reappraise and often reshape the foundations upon which a scientific conditioning program
rests.

Knowledge in the field of exercise physiology is
increased, as it is in other fields, through careful
research. Because of the complexity of the human
organism, exercise physiology research necessitates
a wide range of study. Research findings accrue
largely from two sources: (1) empirical or subjective
observations on large numbers of people of a clinical
case study nature reported from experience by well-
trained professionals, and (2) laboratory studies performed in a controlled environment often utilizing
elaborate and sophisticated instrumentation. These
studies usually involve a few subjects who represent
but a small sample of the total population. Both of
these sources are important in their contribution to
the general knowledge of human performance. Although laboratory studies are preferred because they
provide greater control of the variables being observed, it is often impracticable to study certain factors of a physiological nature under such conditions.
The very nature of some parameters requiring study,
for example, the aging process, make it difficult
to utilize the best experimental laboratory control.
Therefore, subjectively determined data and subse-

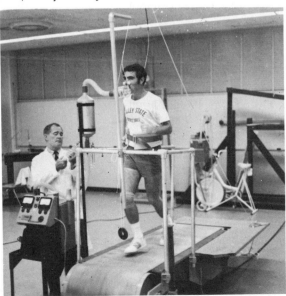

FIGURE 1.2
Laboratory Assessment of
Physical Working Capacity
(Maximum Oxygen
Consumption). The subject
runs to exhaustion on a
treadmill while his expired
air is collected and
analyzed for its oxygen
content (Photo courtesy
of Physical Education
Research Laboratory,
San Fernando Valley
State College).

quently reported findings reinforced by large numbers of investigators serve as an equally valid source of information about certain factors of performance. An illustration of the use of instrumentation in a laboratory setting for the study of cardiorespiratory function is shown in Figure 1.2. Bioelectronic and chemical procedures are being employed while a subject is running on a motor driven treadmill.

A. Circulatory Disturbances

Dr. Paul Dudley White (1957, 1959), an eminent cardiologist, has for many years stressed the hazards of inactivity. His writings touch on our soft way of life and the illness problems which come with prosperity and inactivity. These include obesity, high blood pressure, and atherosclerosis. He feels it has been well-demonstrated that physical fitness lessens the development and effect of these conditions. For example, good muscle tone in the legs helps to supplement the return of blood to the heart thereby improving general circulation of the body. He stresses two important outcomes of vigorous activities. First they serve as an antidote to nervous tension, and second they help the prevention of obesity through increased calorie consumption. Physical fitness of the middle-aged person is the most neglected. Through emphasis on physical activity throughout one's lifetime, problems of advanced age will be lessened. The most likely candidate for coronary atherosclerosis is the obese, heavy smoking, sedentary adult male with a high blood lipid content and high blood pressure (Spain, 1966).

Many other cardiologists are of the opinion that much cardiovascular disease can be prevented through regular physical activity (see Canadian Medical Association, 1967). Additional research confirms that individuals in occupations of a sedentary nature when compared with those in more strenuous occupations have a higher mortality rate. Most of the population studies comparing persons in sedentary and nonsedentary occupations show that, in general, the sedentary individuals who do not participate in regular physical activity have a higher rate of coronary artery disease (Goerke, et al., 1957; Fox and Haskell, 1967; Taylor, 1967; Kannel, 1967). Regular participation in muscular activity has become one of Man's necessary supplemental daily activities if he is to maintain an optimum physiological function of the circulatory mechanism.

B. Connective Tissue Adaptations

Another physiological malfunction which may result from inactivity is adaptive shortening of connective tissue. In certain areas of the body (for example, the lower back) dense connective tissue known as *fascia* has the function of reinforcement of active muscle contraction. This holding action of connective tissue "spells off" the antigravity muscles of the back and serves as an energy conserving mechanism. When the antigravity muscles tire and their burden is borne completely by the heavy connective tissue of the back, this fascia or connective tissue may become adapted to the stress of bearing the weight. A body position that is sustained, as in an increased lower back curve, often results in shortening of these tissues. Once adaptive shortening has occurred, the need for flexibility or increased range of motion becomes evident. Often associated with lack of flexibility is pain, which may result from irritated nerve endings upon movement. This condition occurs not only in the lower back region but in other parts of the body as well. Orthopedic surgeons report that as much as 80 percent of lower back pain may be due to inactivity (Kraus and Raab, 1961). Physicians emphasize that physical activity is essential from a preventive and therapeutic standpoint.

C. Antigravity Musculature

The physical condition of Man's muscles must be such that he can resist adequately the pull of gravity to maintain an erect posture. Since the skeletal framework of the body has a tendency to collapse with the force of gravity, a great deal of energy is spent throughout the day in combating this force through the use of muscles that maintain an upright posture. In other words, Man is almost constantly making an effort to extend the body. Those muscles which maintain extension, the antigravity muscles (Figure 1.3), due to constant activity, tend to become fatigued as one reaches the end of the day. If these muscles are not well-conditioned, they are not equipped to withstand for many hours the stresses imposed upon them by gravity.

The downward pressure of gravity applied to the bones of the skeleton tends to cause it to buckle at three principle points: the ankle, knee and hip. Since the weight of the body is largely in front of the spinal column, the body tends to fall forward. In order to counteract these tendencies toward buckling, a minimum of five muscles or muscle groups must be activated. The muscles involved in the lower limb are the soleus and gastrocnemius (triceps surae) at the ankle, the quadriceps femoris at the knee, and the gluteus maximus at the hip. The trunk is held upright by the erector spinae muscles running from the sacrum to the base of the skull. If these muscles should pull equally from both ends, the trunk would tend to move backward. Therefore, a fifth muscle group, the abdominals serve as reflex antigravity muscles by maintianing the proper relationship between the rib cage and pelvis in the front. Exercises for these antigravity muscles are fundamental to any general conditioning exercise program. In fact, the design of any well-rounded exercise program might well begin with a consideration of this minimally essential musculature.

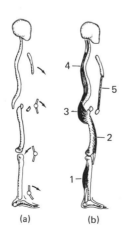

(a)   (b)

FIGURE 1.3
Antero-posterior
Antigravity Musculature
of the Body.
(a) Force of gravity results
in a tendency for the
skeleton to collapse at
points shown by arrows.
(b) Antigravity muscle
groups resist the effect of
gravity and help hold the
body in upright posture.
The muscle groups are:

(1) Triceps surae,
(2) Quadriceps femoris,
(3) Gluteus maximus,
(4) Erector spinae, and
(5) Abdominals (From
Wallis, E. L., and
Logan, G. A. (1964).
*Figure Improvement
and Body Conditioning
through Exercise.*
© 1964. By permission of
Prentice-Hall, Englewood
Cliffs, New Jersey.)

D. Physical Growth

It is important for the adult to be concerned about well-conditioned antigravity muscles, but, perhaps more important, is the need for physical activity in the growth process of children. Vigorous physical activity is essential in order that the child's physical potential may be realized. Rarick (1960) reported that heavy muscular activity in childhood tends to increase lateral growth and vigorously active children tend to have sturdier bodies and maintain a more normal weight than children who are generally sedentary.

The growth of bone has received extensive study since the middle of the 19th century. One of the earliest and perhaps most important results of these efforts was the formulation of Wolff's Law (Sherrington, 1951) which states: "Every change in the form and function of a bone or of their function alone, is followed by certain definite changes in their internal architecture, and equally definite secondary alteration in their external conformation, in accordance with mathematical laws" (Logan, 1964). Later, Steindler (1955) in attempting to adjust for the questionable statement regarding mathematical laws suggested that the internal architecture and the external shape were altered by stresses applied. Mainland (1945), in a research review on the relationship between pressure and bone growth, found that slight continuous pressure often causes atrophy. On the other hand, pressures that are intermittent, including those that are just short of causing trauma, appear to stimulate bone growth. These findings indicate the desirability of participation in strenuous muscular activity during the period of bone growth.

Knipping and Valentin (1961), writing on the concept of function and structure as it relates to growth of muscles and bones, indicated that the kinetic stimulus is indispensible for life and that lack of this stimulus results in underdevelopment. They noted further that stimuli beyond maintenance levels will enhance the organism's ability to respond to greater demands. Lamb (1968) has recently reviewed the subject and presented considerable evidence favoring physical activity as a means of optimally stimulating bone growth and metabolism.

E. Smooth Muscle

The relationship between exercise and the functional efficiency of maintenance systems of the organism has not been studied sufficiently. Of primary concern is the effect of exercise on smooth muscle in the blood vascular system. Most of the evidence in this area is of a clinical nature. Chapman (1959) has pointed out that the only way blood vessels can get exercise is to place a greater demand on the body for oxygen. With this greater demand more blood is pumped through the vessels which then dilate and later constrict. He indicated that this alternate dilation and constriction was exercise, and if these muscles are not exercised they atrophy like other muscles in the body. Although the evidence from scientific studies is quite limited, it appears likely that smooth muscle would become stronger by increasing its work output just as skeletal muscle does.

F. Rest and Sleep

The human organism must be provided with adequate amounts of rest and sleep. Whether or not exercise will aid in the ability to sleep seems to be related to the vigorousness of the activity. In general, it appears that mild exercise tends to promote sleep and that overexertion may interfere with sleep. Although it is possible for the body to go for long periods without sleep—over a week in some experimental cases—experimental study seems to indicate that maximum work performance can be adversely affected (Holland, 1965). Physical activity performed below the level of exhaustion tends to promote a state of "natural" muscular relaxation. This type of relaxation appears beneficial and may be conducive to sleep. The psychological benefits of physical activity, no doubt, play a part in the promotion of sleep.

G. Posture

The contribution of exercise to prevention and correction of body malalignments cannot be overemphasized. Marked deviations in body alignment during the growth years may become more pronounced, persist even into adulthood, and become irreversible. Since a child's malleable bones can be malformed in shape and structure in accordance with Wolff's Law, proper alignment is essential. It is during childhood that corrective measures must be taken. The value of good posture is important from both a physiological and aesthetic viewpoint. Aesthetic standards of posture demand that the individual present himself in an upright, alert, active-looking appearance. Because posture is often the result of mental state, well-conditioned antigravity muscles do not always assure desirable alignment. When a person's attitude is optimistic and he is well, an erect posture is usually evident. In contrast, when he is depressed, dissatisfied, or ill, the characteristics of poor posture are seen. Consequently, the solution of postural problems does not depend on exercise alone. Attitude and inherited bone structure impose limitations that exercise cannot overcome. However, exercise can serve as a valuable therapeutic adjunct.

H. Injury Prevention

There are several ways in which well-developed musculature serves to lessen the incidence of injury. Factors involved in the prevention of bodily injury are strength, endurance, flexibility, and skill. The development of an optimum level of these factors tends to provide a more efficient and skillful function when an injury situation is imminent. Alley (1964), in an extensive study dealing with head and neck injuries received in high school football, reported that where schools had longer preseason programs of conditioning fewer injuries occurred. Most of the reports of contact injuries resulting in sports tend to show that the ankle, knee, and shoulder joints are the most frequent sites of injuries causing disablement and loss of participation time. It is through strengthening of the muscles which support these joints that increased stability occurs. Bender et al. (1964) reported that exercise aided significantly in the prevention of injuries to the knee.

Optimum levels of muscular endurance provide the individual with the ability to sustain activity for a longer period thereby delaying the onset of fatigue. In a fatigued state, the person is apt to react less vigorously than he would if higher levels of endurance had been previously established (Davis et al., 1965). Flexibility of joints or the range through which they can be moved plays a part in the prevention of injury. The stronger the ligaments, the more stability is to be found in the joints. Recent scientific studies indicate that habitual exercise is sufficient to cause a significant increase in the strength of ligaments surrounding and protecting the knee (Adams, 1966; Tipton, et al., 1967; Zuckerman and Stull, 1969). Further study is required but at this point it may be postulated that exercise has a favorable effect on ligament strength, and consequently, corresponding stability of joints.

Improved skill of movement is also an adjunct to the avoidance of injury. In hazardous situations, it appears likely that the more skilled individual would be less accident prone. The development of skill through muscular activity is not only important for the performance of a variety of activities, but also has obvious benefits other than those directly related to the activity being performed.

Another injury preventing outcome of muscular activity is hypertrophy or increased girth of muscle. In some vulnerable areas of the body, this thickened tissue may serve as a form of padding and thereby offer a deterrent to traumatic injury to underlying structures. One who is well-developed muscularly has the advantage of being less susceptible to injury in contact sports. Of particular importance here is the need for development of the trunk and the upper limbs. In almost all reports concerning the incidence of injuries in contact activities, a plea is made for emphasis on the development of the upper body.

I. Rehabilitation

The use of exercise for therapeutic purposes in the rehabilitation of both physical and mental problems is well-established. The development of medical specialists such as the physiatrist, a medical doctor who specializes in physical medicine and rehabilitation, is evidence of the importance of muscular activity as an adjunct to medicine. A variety of therapists who treat patients with exercise function under the pre- scription of a physician. Of course, these therapists use other treatment modalities as well as exercise.

Of particular importance are new developments in the understanding and use of exercise in the re- habilitation of the cardiac patient. Dr. Paul Dudley White is among the leading spokesmen for the use of exercise for this aspect of medical rehabilitation. He has stressed the importance of exercise in the recovery phase after a coronary attack as well as the general benefits of good muscle tone and the value of exercise for mental and physical health throughout the aging process (White, 1957).

J. Tension Relief

Many people use physical activity as a means of re- lease from mental states often commonly referred to as "tension." Emotions are best dissipated in the form of activity. There are several ways in which exercise can provide emotional outlets. These in- clude providing opportunities for creative expres- sion, self-confidence, and achievement (Riedman, 1950). Physical activity as a form of diversion in which the performer becomes "lost" in the activity can provide tension releasing intervals for many in- dividuals. Those who have experienced a mild state of physical fatigue after a pleasant, vigorous bout of exercise can attest to the benefits of "natural" re- laxation during and after the ensuing recovery pe- riod. Too often, this value of exercise is overlooked.

An increasing use of exercise is being made in psychiatry. The role of exercise in psychiatry devel- oped and gained widespread acceptance in the vet- erans' hospitals. Layman (1960) made an extensive review of the application of exercise in psychiatric treatment. It was found that this kind of treatment had far-reaching benefits and may serve where other kinds of treatment are unsuccessful.

K. Aging

The average length of life has doubled in the past century due largely to improved living conditions and the advancement of medical science. An understanding of the aging process is becoming a primary concern from both a sociological and medical standpoint because of increasing numbers of older people. Just as during the growing years aging leads to improvement; in the later years aging appears as deterioration (Karvonen, 1961b). Deterioration is seen in physiological function with an associated increase of degenerative diseases. There is agreement that physical performance is decreased with the passing of time (Bortz, 1960). The findings of Shock (1962) indicate a wide variation and lack of corresponding equal decline among the systems of the body. For example, between the years of 50 and 60, maximum voluntary breathing capacity and kidney plasma flow decrease much more rapidly than the other nine physiological functions studied. He feels that the relationships between organ systems become distorted because of the difference in aging rate of these systems. This would tend to result in incoordination among systems and may explain some of the decrease in physical performance capacity that is noted. Shock concludes that the most noted characteristic of aging is a decrease in the ability of the capacities of the body to return rapidly to a normal level after equilibrium has been disturbed. It has been shown that many of the phenomena of aging seem to be opposite of those which result from the effects of training. Due to this fact physical rehabilitation shows promise of being effective in retarding some of the processes of aging (Karvonen, 1961a).

L. Longevity

The effects of exercise on the length of life have been a subject of study for some time. Most of the studies have been of athletes and nonathletes and their length of life. There is not much difference in the life expectancy of college athletes and nonathletes. However, whether or not men participated in sports in college shows little relationship to the amount of regular and continuous physical activity performed by them in their later years. It is believed that the amount of physical activity in which the person participates throughout his lifetime may be the important factor affecting longevity rather than sports participation in youth (Montoye, 1960). Karvonen (1961b) suggests that exercise throughout life has a positive effect on health because people feel better and function more efficiently in daily living even if exercise does not prolong life.

III. SOME MISCONCEPTIONS ABOUT EXERCISE

In spite of the abundance of evidence concerning the effect and benefits of exercise, there are an astonishing number of misconceptions about its function and use. For example, the idea persists that concentrating on the development of physical fitness among children will result in subsequent adult physical fitness. The physical fitness of children is important because it influences growth and development, but it must be realized that in order to retain physical fitness during adult years, exercise must be employed at appropriate levels and durations commensurate with the individual's tolerance throughout his life span. In other words, the maintenance of physical fitness is an ongoing, persistent necessity that may not be provided by the conditioning of children alone.

Another misconception held by some is that development and subsequent increased size of the normal heart through exercise is harmful. The heart responds to exercise demands just as do the other muscles of the body (Kraus and Raab, 1961). Only by placing demands on this muscle is it possible to increase its functional capacity. Through exercise the heart becomes capable of satisfying the demands for blood imposed by the other systems of the body upon the cardiovascular system. Because of improvement in functional capacity resulting from exercise, the greater the demand for blood in the tissues of the body, the greater becomes the capacity of the heart to meet that demand.

Claims have been made in favor of time consuming systems of exercise that place insufficient demands upon the body. In other words, exercise should be commensurate with the tolerance capacity of the individual. The application of stresses that raise the tolerance capacity of the individual is a judicious utilization of time. Calisthenic-type exercise programs often do not impose adequate levels of stress in proportion to the amount of time spent.

Claims are made asserting the permanent and lasting effects of exercise. Most of the effects of exercise are not permanent. The adjustments made by the body to imposed demands are largely reversible; without continuing demands, capacity diminishes. Functional capacity cannot be retained unless regular activity is maintained.

The misconception continues to persist that deep breathing is a fundamental exercise. It is difficult to conceive of the advantages of such an exercise. A critical analysis of this exercise reveals that the blood is not further oxygenated by forced inspiration, that lung capacity is not greatly increased, and that resistance to respiratory diseases is not developed. On the basis of present knowledge, time spent on such exercise is not justified. Any intentional regulation of breathing rate and rhythm is unnecessary since the breathing apparatus is reflexly, or automatically, regulated by the demands imposed upon it.

There is also a notion that the way in which one breathes during exercise has some influence upon strength development and other fitness factors. There is no substantiation of this belief. Exercise is usually best performed without any conscious attention to breathing. The one exception applies when a maximum effort is made against resistance. When maximum effort is being exerted, the trachea should be kept open as a safety measure to prevent possible harmful effects caused by extreme intra-abdominal and intra-thoracic pressures. These pressures might cause weakened blood vessels to rupture or other types of herniations. During extreme efforts, breathing helps to prevent these possible harmful effects and to prevent the build-up of pressure. Specific breathing exercises may be prescribed for therapeutic purposes, but for those participating in normal conditioning programs, breathing exercises are of little consequence.

Another misconception concerning the function of exercise is that it improves general coordination. Exercise does not specifically facilitate coordination, if coordination is used in terms of the general motor ability to perform skilled acts. However, improvement in strength, endurance, and flexibility may provide the basic essentials upon which skill may be built. In other words, the development of strength, endurance, and flexibility through exercise does not enable the individual to better perform specific coordinations. However, a minimum level of these factors, which can be developed through exercise, is essential as a foundation for the development of specific coordinations.

Finally, contrary to some beliefs, there is no food that has special influence on the development of strength provided that a normal, balanced diet is available. Although it is true that the protein requirements of the body are somewhat greater during periods of growth or rapid strength development, high protein diets are not necessary if "high protein diet" is interpreted to mean more protein than is ordinarily recommended in a basic diet for an active person (Rasch and Pierson, 1962). In addition, fluid intake has little or nothing to do with the development of muscle.

In short, there is no way of developing strength and/or endurance without contracting the muscle under overload conditions.

CHAPTER 1   References

Adams, A. (1966). "Effect of Exercise on Ligament Strength." *Research Quarterly of the American Association for Health, Physical Education, and Recreation* **37**:163–167.

Alley, H. (1964). "Head and Neck Injuries in Football." *Journal American Medical Association* **185** (5):118–122.

Bender, J. A., Kobes, F. J., Kaplan, H. M., and Pierson, J. K. (1964). "Strengthening Muscles and Preventing Injury with a Controlled Program of Isometric Exercises." *Journal of Health, Physical Education, and Recreation* **35**(1):57–58.

Bortz, E. L. (1960). "Exercise, Fitness, and Aging." *In Exercise and Fitness*, pp. 1–9. Athletic Institute, Chicago, Illinois.

Canadian Medical Association (1967). "Proceedings of the International Symposium on Physical Activity and Cardiovascular Health." *Canadian Medical Association Journal* **96**:695–917.

Chapman, A. L. (1959). "The Latest on Exercise and What it Does for You." Copyrighted interview. *United States News and World Report* **XLVI**(23):104–105.

Davis, E. C., Logan, G. A., and McKinney, W. C. (1965). *Biophysical Values of Muscular Activity.* W. C. Brown, Dubuque, Iowa.

Fox, S. M., and Haskell, W. L. (1967). "Population Studies." *Canadian Medical Association Journal* **96**:806–811.

Goerke, L. S., Chapman, J. M., and Phillips, J. E. (1957). "Disease of the Heart in the Working Population: A Study of Morbidity and Mortality in Relation to Cardiac Status and Nature of Job." *California Medicine* **87**:398–401.

Holland, G. (1965). "The Effect of Sleeplessness on Physical Performance." Unpublished doctoral dissertation. University of Southern California, Los Angeles, California.

Kannel, W. B. (1967). "Habitual Level of Physical Activity and Risk of Coronary Heart Disease." *Canadian Medical Association Journal* **96**:811–812.

Karvonen, M. J. (1961a). "Exercise—Physiological Aging." *In Health and Fitness in the Modern World*, pp. 368–370. Athletic Institute, Chicago, Illinois.

Karvonen, M. J. (1961b). "Some Effects of Long Term Exercise on Health and Aging." *In Health and Fitness in the Modern World*, pp. 223–227. Athletic Institute, Chicago, Illinois.

Knipping, H. W., and Valentin, H. (1961). "Sports in Medicine." *In Therapeutic Exercise* (S. Licht, ed.), pp. 354–374. Elizabeth Licht, New Haven.

Kraus, H., and Raab, W. (1961). *Hypokinetic Disease.* Thomas, Springfield, Illinois.

Lamb, D. R. (1968). "Influence of Exercise on Bone Growth and Metabolism." *In Kinesiology Review 1968*, pp. 43–48. American Association for Health, Physical Education, and Recreation, Washington, D.C.

Layman, E. (1960). "Physical Activity as a Psychiatric Adjunct." *In Science and Medicine of Exercise and Sports* (W. R. Johnson, ed.), pp. 703–725. Harper, New York.

Logan, G. A. (1964). *Adaptations of Muscular Activity.* Wadsworth, Belmont, California.

Mainland, D. (1945). *Anatomy as a Basis for Medical and Dental Practice.* Harper, New York.

Montoye, H. (1960). "Sports and Length of Life." *In Science and Medicine of Exercise and Sports* (W. R. Johnson, ed.), pp. 517–522. Harper, New York.

Rarick, G. L. (1960). "Exercise and Growth." *In Science and Medicine of Exercise and Sports* (W. R. Johnson, ed.), pp. 440–465. Harper, New York.

Rasch, P. J., and Pierson, W. R. (1962). "The Effect of a Protein Dietary Supplement on Muscular Strength and Hypertrophy." *American Journal Clinical Nutritian* **11**:530–532.

Riedman, S. R. (1950). *Physiology of Work and Play.* Holt, New York.

Sherrington, C. (1951). *Man on His Nature.* Cambridge University Press, London and New York.

Shock, N. W. (1962). "The Physiology of Aging." *Scientific American* **206**(1):100–110.

Spain, D. M. (1966). "Atherosclerosis." *Scientific American* **215**(2):48–56.

Steindler, A. (1955). *Kinesiology of the Human Body.* Thomas, Springfield, Illinois.

Taylor, H. L. (1967). "Occupational Factors in the Study of Coronary Heart Disease and Physical Activity." *Canadian Medical Association Journal* **96**:825–831.

Tipton, C. M., Schild, R. J., and Tomanek, R. J. (1967). "Influence of Physical Activity on the Strength of Knee Ligaments in Rats." *American Journal Physiology* **212**:783–787.

Wallis, E. L., and Logan, G. A. (1964). *Figure Improvement and Body Conditioning Through Exercise.* Prentice-Hall, Englewood Cliffs, New Jersey.

Wells, K. F. (1966). *Kinesiology.* Saunders, Philadelphia, Pennsylvania.

White, P. D. (1957). "The Role of Exercise in the Aging." *Journal American Medical Association* **165** (1):70–71.

White, P. D. (1959). "The Advantages of Physical Fitness." *Illinois Medical Journal* **116:** 185–187.

Zuckerman, J., and Stull, G. A. (1969). "Effects of Exercise on Knee Ligament Separation in Rats." *Journal Applied Physiology* **26:**716–719.

TWO/ Neuromuscular Mechanisms

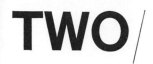

TWO/

Human movement is produced by the force of muscular contraction transmitted to the bones, similar to a mechanical system of articulated levers. Muscle fibers are supplied with nerves which control their activity. When nerve impulses originating in the central nervous system reach the muscle fibers, the fibers contract forcefully. When the impulses cease, the fibers relax. The selection of the specific muscles and muscle fibers and the grading of the force of contraction needed to perform a coordinated act is remarkably complex. The elements of skillful performance, although not completely understood as yet, are more comprehensible now than ever before. Anatomists, kinesiologists, physiologists, molecular biologists, and other specialists in related sciences have produced research during the past two decades which has advanced our understanding of the neuromuscular mechanism and its adaptations.

I. THE CENTRAL NERVOUS SYSTEM AND MOVEMENT

The central nervous system consists of the brain, spinal cord, and 31 pairs of peripheral nerves which branch out from the spinal cord to serve all parts of the body (Figure 2.1). The structural unit of the central nervous system is the nerve cell or *neuron* (Figure 2.2). Billions of these basic cells are interconnected in various ways to form the central nervous system. In addition to the cell body, the typical neuron has extensions, or projections, called *axons* and *dendrites*. The dendrites are a number of short fibers that always conduct the nerve impulses toward the cell body. Axons conduct the impulses away from the cell body. As a result, an impulse traveling through the neuron in Figure 2.2 would progress from the top to the bottom.

Axons are usually much longer than dendrites, some measuring up to three feet in length. Each neuron has only one axon, but it may have several dendrites. Axons make functional connections (*synapses*) with the dendrites of other neurons or terminate in effector organs, for example, muscles. In addition to being longer than dendrites, the axons of some neurons have a fatty covering called the *myelin sheath* (Figure 2.2). Axons having this sheath transmit impulses more rapidly than those without it. Rapid transmission of impulses has significance in the rate at which muscle fibers can be stimulated to contract.

Although one neuron is practically indistinguishable from another in appearance, they are classified according to the manner in which they transmit impulses. They may act as an input pathway to the

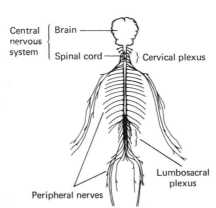

Central nervous system {
Brain
Spinal cord
} Cervical plexus

Lumbosacral plexus

Peripheral nerves

FIGURE 2.1
Schematic Dorsal View of the Central Nervous System. The brain together with some of the principal peripheral nerve roots and nerve trunks are roughly indicated. The entire system is, of course, far more extensive than this diagram shows (From Easton, D. M. *Mechanisms of Body Functions.* © 1963. By permission of Prentice-Hall, Englewood Cliffs, New Jersey.)

central nervous system, as an output pathway from it, or as a connector between input and output. The neurons which act as input mechanisms are termed *sensory* or *afferent* neurons. They receive stimuli from the environment such as light, pressure, odor, etc., convert these to chemical–electrical signals, and transmit them either to the brain or spinal cord. The 31 pairs of spinal nerves transmit impulses to the cord, while the cranial nerves (vision, smell, etc.) transmit impulses directly to the brain. The neurons which act as output mechanisms are termed *motor* or *efferent* neurons. They carry action impulses from the central nervous system causing muscles to contract. Connecting (*association* or *internuncial*) neurons receive impulses from sensory neurons and transfer them to the proper motor neurons for action. The nervous system acts in much the same manner as a telephone communication system. The spinal cord acts as a switchboard, switching incoming impulses from sensory nerve cells to the proper circuit so that they may travel out on motor neurons.

In describing the structural unit of the central nervous system (neuron), the basic functional unit, the *reflex arc*, has also been described. In its simplest form, the reflex arc consists of one sensory neuron which synapses directly with one motor neuron. This simple loop has five essential elements:

(1) *Receptor:* specialized sensory nerve ending which receives information from the environment.

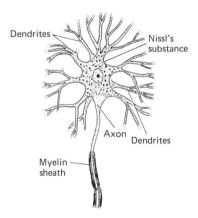

Dendrites

Nissl's substance

Axon Dendrites

Myelin sheath

FIGURE 2.2
A Neuron—Basic Structural Unit of the Nervous System. Networks of this basic cell make up the tissue structures of the entire system (From Wyburn, G. M. (1960). *The Nervous System.* New York: Academic Press).

(2) *Afferent neuron:* the sensory transmitter of impulses from the receptor to the spinal cord.
(3) *Synapse:* connection between the sensory and the motor neuron.
(4) *Efferent neuron:* motor neuron conducting the impulse from the spinal cord to an effector.
(5) *Effector:* organ responsible for response (Singer, 1968).

Figure 2.3 presents a classic example of the simple reflex arc, the knee jerk reflex. When the patellar tendon from the quadriceps muscles is tapped, the resulting stretch effect is picked up by the proprioceptive receptor endings and conducted to the spinal cord. A motor impulse results causing a contraction in the quadriceps muscles to relieve the stretch.

The reflex arc often is of a more complicated nature than in Figure 2.3 involving interconnections with many association and motor neurons. This situation is illustrated in Figure 2.4 where the barefoot individual has stepped on a tack.

A. Muscle—Nerve Relationships

The central nervous system acts as the controlling influence on muscle activity, and each muscle action is the result of one or more impulses sent along the motor neurons from the central nervous system. These muscle actions range from simple reflexes to

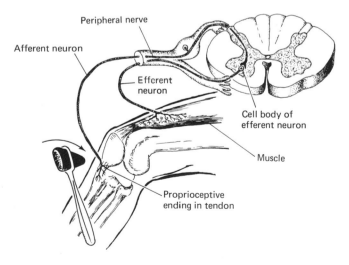

Peripheral nerve

Afferent neuron

Efferent neuron

Cell body of efferent neuron

Muscle

Proprioceptive ending in tendon

FIGURE 2.3
A Simple Reflex Arc (Knee Jerk). Four fundamental parts of a reflex arc are shown: (1) a receptor—proprioceptive ending in tendon; (2) a sensory transmitter—the afferent neuron; (3) a motor transmitter—the efferent neuron; (4) the effector—the muscle (From Grollman, S. *The Human Body.* © 1964. By permission of Macmillan, New York.)

those which involve volitional control, interpretation of patterns, and memory.

1. EXCITABLE TISSUE

The ease with which information travels back and forth between the muscles and the central nervous system is due to the fact that both muscle and nerve are *excitable* tissues. Being excitable means that the tissue is capable of transmitting electrical impulses along its membrane. Impulses transmitted in this way are initiated by various mechanisms. They are generated by touch, light, heat, cold, and so on, or they may be started volitionally by activity within the brain. In nerve tissue the impulse is merely trans-

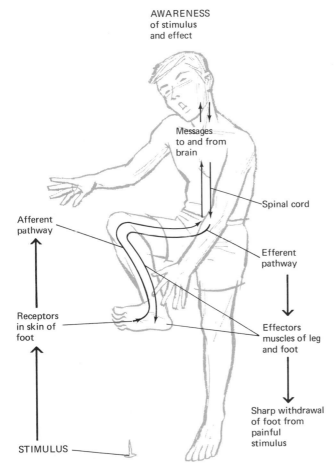

AWARENESS
of stimulus
and effect

Messages
to and from
brain

Spinal cord

Afferent
pathway

Efferent
pathway

Receptors
in skin of
foot

Effectors
muscles of leg
and foot

Sharp withdrawal
of foot from
painful
stimulus

STIMULUS

FIGURE 2.4
Reflex Action
Demonstrating
Many Reflex Arcs
(From McNaught, A.
and Callander, R.
Illustrated Physiology.
© 1963. Williams & Wilkins,
Baltimore, Maryland.
By permission of E. & S.
Livingstone, Ltd., London.)

mitted, in muscle tissue the impulse causes a contraction to occur.

Impulses may travel along muscle and nerve membranes because of the electrical arrangement of ions (a mineral with an electrical charge) on either side of the membranes. In the resting state positively and negatively charged ions are found both inside and outside the membrane. The relative concentration of the two types of ions is different on the inside and outside of the membrane. The inside of the resting cell is negatively charged in contrast with the outside (Figure 2.5b). The membrane is thus said to be polarized with a resting potential of −85 millivolts. This means that the inside of the membrane is 85 millivolts more negative than the outside.

The ion primarily responsible for this situation is sodium (Na+). Some mechanism, as yet incompletely identified, continually transports sodium from the cell. The mechanism is commonly referred to as the *sodium pump*. The sodium pump maintains a greater concentration of sodium ions outside the cell which sustains the membrane potential of −85 millivolts.

When the cell is stimulated the sodium pump somehow becomes less operative, and sodium ions rush into the interior of the cell reversing the membrane potential so that the interior of the cell becomes positive in relation to the outside. This is

FIGURE 2.5
Propagation of Impulse through Excitable Tissue. The action potential wave (a) spreads along the surface of a nerve fiber (b). During the resting state sodium ions (Na) are kept out of the fiber by the "sodium pump." During the rise of the action potential, sodium ions enter the fiber and potassium ions (K) leave it. This reverses the membrane potential and propagates the impulse (From Katz, B. "The Nerve Impulse." *Scientific American* **187**(5):55–64. Copyright © November, 1952 by Scientific American. All rights reserved.)

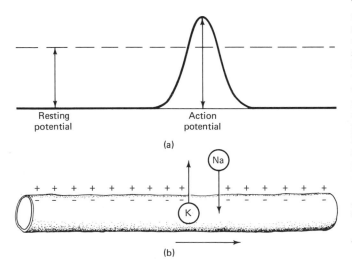

Resting potential   Action potential

(a)

(b)

called *depolarization* and can be recorded as an impulse called the *action potential*. The action potential travels the entire length of the membrane in a self-propagating, wavelike pattern (Figure 2.5a).

As soon as the action potential occurs, immediate reestablishment of the resting potential begins. This is called *repolarization* and is accomplished by diffusion of potassium ions (K^+) out of the cell. This is followed by a renewal of sodium pump activity (Figure 2.5).

2. MOTOR UNITS

A motor unit consists of a nerve fiber and all the muscle fibers with which it connects through its various branches. Figure 2.6 is a schematic representation of a motor unit. Some motor nerves connect with hundreds of muscle fibers in large muscles while other motor units involve very few fibers in the smaller muscles in which finer control is required. Each muscle—nerve trunk combination contains many motor units. A motor nerve impulse causes all of the muscle fibers with which it connects to contract together. A motor unit follows the "all or nothing" principle. There is never a less than maximum contraction of a muscle fiber. *A less than maximum contraction of a whole muscle is achieved by contraction in only a few of the available motor units.* The smoothness of a muscle contraction is accomplished by asynchronous "firing" of motor units. If the muscle fibers involved in a contraction attempt-

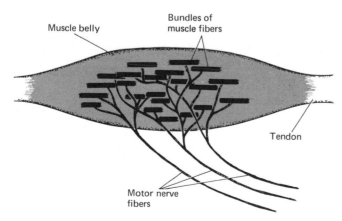

Muscle belly

Bundles of muscle fibers

Tendon

Motor nerve fibers

FIGURE 2.6
Motor Units. This schematic drawing of a muscle shows the distribution of nerve fibers supplying three motor units (From Guyton, A. C. (1964). *Function of the Human Body* (2nd ed.), p. 226. Saunders, Philadelphia, Pennsylvania.)

ed to maintain the contraction indefinitely, they would soon fatigue. Therefore, they must alternately contract and relax in order to be effective. While one group of motor units is relaxing, another group "fires" (contracts). This assures the smoothness of total muscle contraction in most cases.

II. THEORY OF MUSCLE CONTRACTION

Utilizing the electron microscope, H. E. Huxley and his co-workers have conducted experiments in an effort to understand the phenomenon of muscular contraction. These experiments are considered classics in this field of study. These investigations led him to hypothesize the "sliding filament" model of muscle contraction (Huxley, 1958, 1965; Huxley and Hanson, 1960). Electromicrographs show what appear to be tiny filaments within each muscle fiber, the *myofibrils*. During contraction these filaments appear to slide past each other. Figure 2.7 is a schematic representation of how these filaments are arranged in relation to the intact muscle. Figure 2.7 (f) shows the basic unit of contraction, the *sarcomere*. It can be seen in (d) that the sarcomeres are arranged in series along the entire length of the myofibril. Figure 2.8 schematically demonstrates the behavior of a single sarcomere during contraction. Shortening of the sarcomeres occurs along the entire length of the myofibril thereby also shortening the fiber itself. The shortening of several fibers simultaneously causes the muscle to contract resulting in joint movement.

The precise elements involved in inducing the sliding action of the filaments during contraction are not well understood (Rodahl and Horvath, 1960). Most available evidence supports Huxley's view that the thin filaments are composed of the protein actin and the thick ones of the protein myosin. Huxley, as well as most other muscle physiologists, believes there is an interaction between the two via "cross bridges," thus causing actin filaments to "slide" past the myosin filaments. It is believed that the energy for this interaction is provided by the splitting of the phosphagens, adenosine triphosphate and creatine phosphate (Huxley and Hanson, 1960; Rasch and Burke, 1967; Asmussen, 1968; Margaria, 1968). This phosphagen splitting is apparently triggered by the release of acetylcholine at the junction between the nerve and the muscle fibers it stimulates (neuromuscular junction). Acetylcholine is then

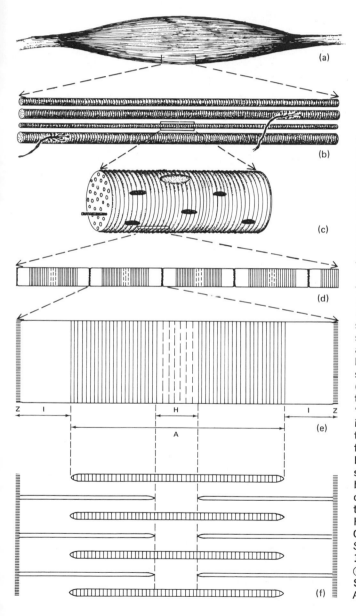

(a)

(b)

(c)

(d)

(e)

(f)

FIGURE 2.7
Skeletal Muscle is Dissected in These Schematic Drawings. A muscle (a) is made up of muscle fibers (b) which appear striated in the light microscope. The small branching structures at the surface of the fibers are the "end-plates" of motor nerves which signal the fibers to contract. A single muscle fiber (c) is made up of myofibrils. In a single myofibril (d) the striations are resolved into a repeating pattern of light and dark bands. A single unit of this pattern (e) consists of a "Z-line," then an "I-band," then an "A-band," which is interrupted by an "H-zone," then the next I-band, and finally the next Z-line. Electron micrographs have shown that the repeating band pattern is due to the overlapping of thick and thin filaments (f) (From Huxley, H. E. "The Contraction of Muscle." *Scientific American* **199**(5):67–82. Copyright © November, 1958 by Scientific American. All rights reserved.)

resynthesized by part of the energy produced in the phosphagen splitting.

The supply of phosphagen in the muscles is small, and it is soon exhausted. Fortunately, the split mole-cules can be resynthesized to provide a continuation

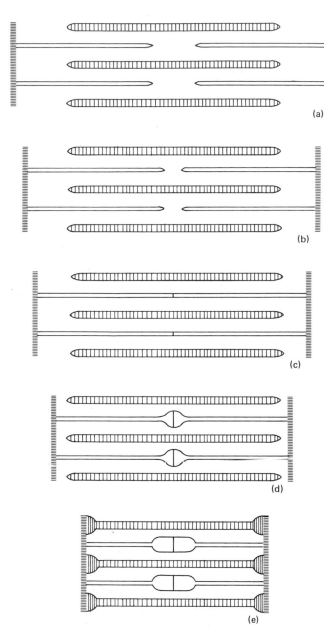

(a)

(b)

(c)

(d)

(e)

FIGURE 2.8
Sliding Filament Model of Muscle Contraction. Change in length of the muscle changes the arrangements of the filaments. In (a) the muscle is stretched; in (b) it is at its resting length; in (c), (d), and (e) it is contracted (From Huxley, H. E. "The Contraction of Muscle." *Scientific American* **199**(5):67–82. © November, 1958 by Scientific American. All rights reserved.)

of the energy producing reactions. The processes involved in this resynthesis are discussed in more detail in Chapter Six.

III. BODY MECHANICS

A. Muscles, Bones, and Joints

The soft tissues of the body (muscle, skin, stomach, intestines, blood vessels, heart, lungs, and so on) are supported by the bony skeletal framework. The segments of this framework are coupled at their ends by articulatory processes called *joints*. Movement of a segment or of the entire body is accomplished by moving parts of the bony framework by contracting some muscles as other muscles relax. The joints allow the bony segments to bend and turn in various directions and ways.

Figure 2.9 depicts the typical interrelationships among bones, joints, and muscles within the body. This illustration presents the arm and shoulder area of the human anatomy. Three of the large bones in this part of the body are schematically shown. At the joints the bones are connected to each other by bands of connective tissue called *ligaments*.

The biceps brachii and the brachialis, large muscles on the anterior portion of the upper arm,

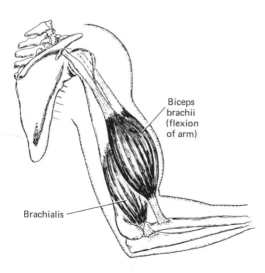

Biceps brachii (flexion of arm)

Brachialis

FIGURE 2.9
Anatomy of the Upper Arm and Shoulder. Shown are the shoulder and elbow joints, the bones involved, and two of the large muscles which flex the elbow. Note how their tendons cross the joints to create a force arm for the lever systems (From Easton, D. M. *Mechanisms of Body Functions.* © 1963. By permission of Prentice-Hall, Englewood Cliffs, New Jersey).

are shown to illustrate the typical relationship between bones, joints, and muscles. The muscle is connected either directly to the bone by its fibers or by an extension of connective tissue from the fibers (the tendon). The tendons cross joints and attach to adjacent bones. One of the muscles shown here, biceps brachii, has tendons which cross two joints. Usually a muscle crosses only one joint. When the muscle contracts (shortens) a pull is applied to the adjacent bone through the tendon. This causes the bone to rotate around its pivotal point at the joint. Thus a body segment moves.

B. Types of Muscle Action

All muscles function by developing or releasing tension. However, the same muscle may vary from time to time in its specific role depending upon the type of action desired in various body segments. There are four basic roles that a muscle or muscle group may perform. The specific role depends upon the requirements of the situation. (1) The muscles which perform the desired action at a given joint are called the *muscles most involved*. (2) The muscles located on the opposite side of the joint or the body part from the muscles most involved are called the *contralateral muscles*. (3) In cases where muscles are located on either side of the muscles most involved and the contralateral musculature, these muscles are called the *guiding muscles*. (4) Muscles that fixate or hold a joint or a body part so that other body parts or joints can move are known as *stabilizing muscles* (Logan and McKinney, 1970).

In Figure 2.9, the pictured muscles would be classified as *muscles most involved*. The triceps brachii, which is located on the posterior part of the upper arm, is a *contralateral muscle* during the movement shown (elbow flexion). In elbow extension against resistance (opposite movement to flexion), the triceps brachii would become the *muscle most involved*, and the biceps brachii and brachialis *contralateral muscles*. The muscles in the shoulder area (not shown here), which attach to the bone of the upper arm, act as *stabilizing muscles* in both cases.

IV. CONTROL OF MOVEMENT

A. Proprioception

Awareness of body position is determined by a variety of sensory inputs to the central nervous system. The organs of balance in the inner ear, vision, and pressures applied to the surface of the body help to provide information on the position of the body and its segments. The muscles and joints are provided with special organs to sense position and tension within the muscles and in the joints. These sensory receptors are known as *proprioceptors* (Granit, 1955). *Muscle spindles* and *Golgi tendon organs* are the major structures involved in proprioception. Muscle spindles are specialized muscle fibers (intrafusal fibers) distributed between some of the contractile fibers in skeletal muscles. Golgi tendon organs are sensory receptors located between the fibers of the muscle tendon. Both of these special structures can initiate the sensory input associated with a reflex arc.

The muscle spindle is sensitive to changes in length and tension of muscle fibers. When the fibers are stretched, the muscle spindle is also stretched, and an impulse is generated which carries this information to the spinal cord. This incoming impulse causes a motor neuron with which it synapses to "fire" resulting in contraction of muscle fibers to oppose the muscle stretch. At the same time impulses travel through a separate motor neuron which causes contraction in the intrafusal muscle fiber to reset the spindle at a new length coinciding with the new contracted length of the surrounding skeletal muscle fibers. This basic mechanism is illustrated in Figure 2.10. This reflex is called the *stretch (myotatic) reflex*. The spindle facilitates the contraction of the muscle surrounding it.

The Golgi tendon organ functions somewhat differently from the muscle spindle. Although it too is sensitive to stretch, it operates as a sensor of high tension on the muscle tendon. When there is a possibility that the muscle tendon will become overloaded as a result of strong muscle contractions, it causes an *antimyotatic* reflex which inhibits contraction in the muscle most involved and often in the contralateral muscles also. This reflex acts as a protective mechanism for the involved joints and muscles. Figure 2.3 presents a classic example of the antimyotatic reflex, the knee jerk reflex.

There are many other proprioceptive receptors located in various parts of the body. They are located in joints, muscles, and in close proximity to other body organs. Their major function is to provide the central nervous system with an awareness of the body and its segments in relation to time and space. The semicircular canals of the inner ear are an example of these other proprioceptors.

B. Volitional Control of Muscle Movement

Voluntary control of movement is caused by impulses originating in the cerebral cortex of the brain. Figure 2.1 presents the brain in relation to other portions of the central nervous system. Figure 2.11 illustrates the part of the brain called the *cerebrum.* The motor, premotor, and somesthetic (sensory)

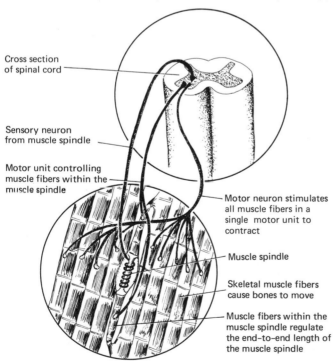

Cross section of spinal cord

Sensory neuron from muscle spindle

Motor unit controlling muscle fibers within the muscle spindle

Motor neuron stimulates all muscle fibers in a single motor unit to contract

Muscle spindle

Skeletal muscle fibers cause bones to move

Muscle fibers within the muscle spindle regulate the end-to-end length of the muscle spindle

FIGURE 2.10
A Muscle Spindle (From Wallis, E. L., and Logan, G. A. *Figure Improvement and Body Conditioning Through Exercise.* © 1964. By permission of Prentice-Hall, Englewood Cliffs, New Jersey).

portions of the cortex are shaded. Many large ascending and descending tracts of neurons have their termination or origin in these areas. The sensory terminations for proprioception, vision, smell, touch, taste, hearing, and so on, are located in the somesthetic area. Sensory input fibers bring information to this localized area of the brain. It should be noted that some sensory fibers terminate in the cerebellum and the midbrain as well.

Descending tracts of fibers originate in both the motor and premotor areas of the cerebral cortex. However, branches and interconnections also go to the midbrain, cerebellum, and somesthetic area of the cerebral cortex. Motor impulses initiating specific movements apparently arise in the motor area and impulses for *patterns of movement* originate in the premotor area (de Vries, 1966). Figure 2.12 is a schematic illustration of one of these descending pathways of nerve fibers as it progresses from the cerebrum through the midbrain, pons, medulla, and segments of the spinal cord.

The exact manner in which the brain "memorizes" a skilled movement for later recall is unknown. Within the large pool of neurons available, the skill is engraved in patterns called *engrams*. There is evidence to indicate that these engrams may be patterned in any one of four areas: the premotor, the motor, the somesthetic, or the basal ganglia of the midbrain. The determination of the location of a

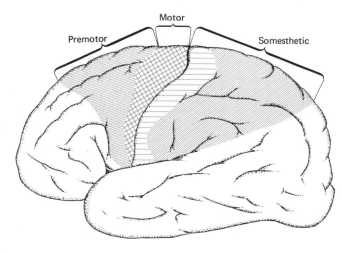

FIGURE 2.11
The Cerebral Cortex. The motor, premotor, and somesthetic areas are shaded (From Guyton, A. C. (1966). *Textbook of Medical Physiology*, p. 802, Saunders, Philadelphia, Pennsylvania).

specific engram is unknown. There is a possibility that the complexity of the skill is a factor in the specific site of memorization (Guyton, 1966; Singer, 1968; de Vries, 1966).

C. Coordination of Muscle Action and Motor Learning

Although the motor impulses originate in the motor and premotor areas (Figure 2.11), research has shown that many areas of the brain are involved in coordinating a motor act. The degree of involvement of specific brain areas is dependent on the specific motor act and the complexity of it. The cerebellum apparently functions as an integrating mechanism in the control of voluntary movements (Snider, 1958; Guyton, 1966).

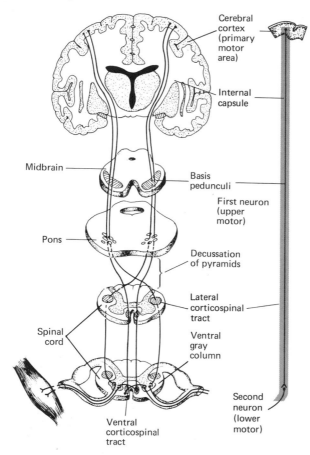

FIGURE 2.12
Pyramidal Motor Pathways, the Corticospinal Tracts. The tracts originate in pyramidal cells of the cerebral cortex. They descend through segments of the brain and spinal cord until they synapse with lower motor neurons connecting to muscles (From Langley, L. L., Telford, I. R., and Christensen, J. B. (1969). *Dynamic Anatomy and Physiology*. Reprinted with permission of McGraw-Hill, New York).

Figure 2.13 is a schematic illustration of the pathways involved in a motor act. The major structures involved are the motor cortex, cerebellum, muscles, red nucleus and thalamus of the midbrain, and reticular formation (neuron pools) of the brain stem and midbrain. The interconnecting pathways among these structures are also illustrated.

When motor impulses are transmitted downward from the cerebral cortex through the corticospinal tract of Figure 2.12, collateral impulses are transmitted simultaneously into the cerebellum. This makes the cerebellum aware of the signals that are sent to the muscles. As the muscles respond to these signals, impulses from the peripheral proprioceptive receptors are sent back to the cerebellum through the spinocerebellar tract. This makes the cerebellum

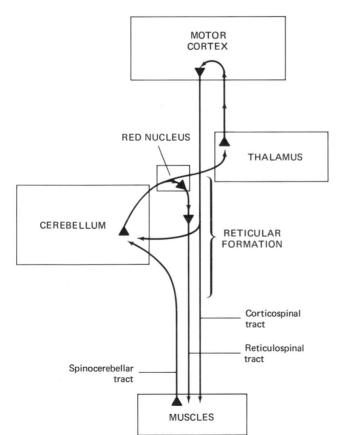

FIGURE 2.13
Pathways for Cerebellar "Error" Control of Voluntary Movements (From Guyton, A. C. (1966). *Textbook of Medical Physiology*, p. 811. Saunders, Philadelphia, Pennsylvania).

aware of what the muscles are actually doing in response to the signals from the motor cortex. The cerebellum is thus able to make a rapid comparison of the "intentions" of the cortex with the "performance" of the muscles.

If the "intentions" and the "performance" do not coincide, the cerebellum is able to effect an adjustment *before* the movement is completed by sending impulses via the red nucleus to the muscles and through both the red nucleus and thalamus to the motor cortex (Figure 2.13). This function of the cerebellum is called *error control* and is very important in skilled movement (Snider, 1958; Guyton, 1966). It should be noted that fast movements, once started, cannot be altered, but adjustments can be made in succeeding movements (Hubbard, 1960).

D. Motor Learning

Many scientists look upon the nervous system as being analogous to an electronic computer. They believe that organized memory traces (engrams) may be stored in the brain in much the same manner that information is stored in various circuits in the computer. When sensory data enters the nervous system, the appropriate program is selected and activated with the electrical impulses passing through a specific set of predetermined circuits (neurons). The specific set of circuits would depend upon the circumstances and how well the skill has been learned. The various programs become effective and efficient with repetition (practice). Practice aids in effecting the process of inhibiting unwanted or extraneous circuits and facilitating the desired ones.

The reticular formation has been termed the program-selection area of the brain (Singer, 1968). As a response selector, the reticular system assigns priorities to messages, determines which are important, and selects appropriate responses in order of importance. This brain area is able to effectively do this because nearly all incoming and outgoing impulses pass through it.

When a skill is conditioned the act must be repeated many times until there develops an automatic association between sensory input and the correct motor response. With practice there is a freer flow of impulses due to repetition. This is known as *neural facilitation*. Repetition reinforces the connection between stimulus and response. In learning a sports skill one must establish a series of conditioned reflexes. These are built up through practice into connections with stored past experiences.

V. THE SAID PRINCIPLE

As Steggerda (1960) most aptly put it, "I am fit to do things that you cannot do because of the type of physical activities I have forced my nervous system to adjust to." The body responds rather specifically to demands placed on it. This is a unifying principle that applies to any of the characteristics that comprise physical fitness. The concept is called the *SAID* principle. The word has been coined from the first letter in the phrase: "Specific Adaptations to *Imposed Demands*" (Wallis and Logan, 1964). This principle provides a general guide to the design of an exercise program. Application of the SAID principle leads to an efficient application of exercise stresses. The principle is justified in theory and supported by much research and careful observation. In order to obtain results from an exercise program *the demands must be sufficient to force adaptation.* It is hypothesized that much, if not all, of the adaptation is basically neurological.

The nerve—muscle relationships described previously are involved in the development of strength, endurance, flexibility, and skill. If, during a period of progressive conditioning, the nervous system is continually forced by tension in the muscle to respond with heightened motor output, the skeletal muscle is "trained" to exert more force because the neural function begins to operate with more facility. The impulses flow more freely than before. This phenomenon is known as *neural facilitation,* and it is a major factor in motor learning. This is the neurological basis for explaining the SAID principle. Using strength as an example, it can be seen that increased ability of the muscle to exert force is dependent upon imposing demands that will result in neural facilitation.

Therefore, it might be said that the body learns to be strong through practice in working the muscles against resistance. And the "learning" is rather specific. One may "learn" to use muscles strongly in certain ways and in certain coordinations, but he may find other tasks utilizing the same musculature to be more difficult than would be anticipated. Again, the SAID principle applies.

It should be understood that in addition to neurological factors the broader physiological "base" for muscular strength is also elevated through training. That is, the ability to withstand fatigue and generate force is dependent upon adequate oxygen supply and nutritional elements stored within and made available to the contractile tissue. These factors will be discussed in greater detail later. Internal chemical condition and the training of "latent" fibers are involved in improving functional ability. This improved chemical—nutritional foundation can be made to function more efficiently through heightened levels of neural stimulation.

The development of endurance involves a similar neurological basis to that of strength development. Some types of localized endurances result from the continued facilitation of the same mechanisms already described. In addition, endurance involves the elevation of the general base—greater output of the heart muscle, the opening of more capillaries, improved oxygen-carrying capacity of the blood, and other related training effects which are basic adaptations.

An increase in the range of motion of the joints of the body also has a basis in neurological function. Flexibility results from stretching the membranes that surround muscles, stretching tendons, and lengthening the ligaments and other tissues that limit the movement of the joint.

As the muscle on one side of a joint shortens, the muscle on the other side lengthens. To stretch an area there must be a relaxation of the muscles in the area. Without this relaxation the muscle tends to resist the stretching action. As the muscles on one side of the joint are contracted, the muscles on the other side are reciprocally inhibited. Therefore, contracting the muscles opposite the area being stretched provides the favorable conditions for lengthening the connective tissue that surrounds the muscle.

When attempting to increase flexibility through stretching, reflex muscle contraction tends to limit the range of motion as a self-protecting mechanism. To minimize this reflex activity in the area being stretched, slow, sustained contractions of the muscles opposite are preferable to rapid movements involving momentum. This causes a slow firing of the muscle spindles and is less likely to result in injury.

From the above examples it becomes obvious that demands placed upon the organism by exercise must be sufficient to force adaptation. Therefore, exercise that is too mild is nearly valueless and is a waste of time from a conditioning standpoint. The one major principle, SAID, through which improvement of fitness, bodily function, and form may be achieved, involves placing the body under stresses of varying intensity and duration. By attempting to overcome these stresses the body adapts rather specifically to these imposed demands and, as a result, elevates the tolerance for further activity of greater intensity. Since individual tolerance for exercise varies, it becomes necessary to have gradation or progression in the intensity or severity of the exercise. This principle of pushing the systems to force their development of endurance, flexibility, and strength is the theme of this book. It goes a step further in attempting to provide the reader with a background for understanding the physiology and anatomy of adaptations that are made in response to the imposed demands.

CHAPTER 2 References

Asmussen, E. (1968). "The Neuromuscular System and Exercise." In Exercise Physiology (H. B. Falls, ed.), pp. 3–42. Academic Press, New York.

de Vries, H. A. (1966). Physiology of Exercise for Physical Education and Athletics. W. C. Brown, Dubuque, Iowa.

Granit, R. (1955). *Receptors and Sensory Perception.* Yale University Press, New Haven, Connecticut.

Guyton, A. C. (1966). *Textbook of Medical Physiology.* Saunders, Philadelphia, Pennsylvania.

Hubbard, A. W. (1960). "Homokinetics: Muscular Function in Human Movement." *In Science and Medicine of Exercise and Sports* (W. R. Johnson, ed.), pp. 7–39. Harper, New York.

Huxley, H. E. (1958). "The Contraction of Muscle." *Scientific American* **199**(5):67–82.

Huxley, H. E. (1965). "The Mechanism of Muscular Contraction." *Scientific American* **213**(6):18–27.

Huxley, H. E., and Hanson, J. (1960). "The Molecular Basis of Contraction in Cross-striated Muscles." *In Structure and Function of Muscle,* Vol. I (G. H. Bourne, ed.), pp. 183–228. Academic Press, New York.

Logan, G. A., and McKinney, W. C. (1970). *Kinesiology: Analysis of Sport and Exercise.* W. C. Brown, Dubuque, Iowa.

Margaria, R. (1968). "Energy Sources for Aerobic and Anaerobic Work." *In Physiological Aspects of Sports and Physical Fitness* (B. Balke, ed.), pp. 20–25. Athletic Institute, Chicago, Illinois.

Rasch, P. J., and Burke, R. K. (1967). *Kinesiology and Applied Anatomy.* Lea & Febiger, Philadelphia, Pennsylvania.

Rodahl, K., and Horvath, S. M. (eds.) (1960). *Muscle as a Tissue,* pp. 63–160. McGraw-Hill, New York.

Singer, R. N. (1968). *Motor Learning and Human Performance.* Macmillan Company, New York.

Snider, R. S. (1958). "The Cerebellum." *Scientific American* **199**(2):84–94.

Steggerda, F. R. (1960). "The Role of the Nervous System in Fitness." *In Exercise and Fitness,* pp. 68–72. Athletic Institute, Chicago, Illinois.

Wallis, E. L., and Logan, G. A. (1964). *Figure Improvement and Body Conditioning through Exercise.* Prentice-Hall, Englewood Cliffs, New Jersey.

THREE / Flexibility

THREE/

I. BASIS FOR FLEXIBILITY

Inactive people usually are inflexible. Sedentary living habits and the habitual use of the flexor apparatus of the body are often major reasons for lack of sufficient range of motion or flexibility. Lacking sufficient activity to stimulate the maintenance of the antigravity muscles of the body and using mainly the flexor muscles necessitates the use of flexibility exercises for certain areas. These areas are the posterior thigh, anterior hip, low back, neck, and the pectoral area of the chest.

A reasonable degree of flexibility is required for sufficient bodily function. In order for the muscles to move the bony levers, the muscles opposite those performing the movement (contralateral muscles) must lengthen sufficiently. Ligamentous joint structures and other connective tissue also restrict the range of motion since inactivity causes these tissues to lose their extensibility. If complete range of motion does not exist, it can be regained through judiciously applied flexibility exercises.

There seems to be some difference in the natural degree of flexibility possessed by various people. Some have shorter muscles, some have shorter ligaments, and some have bodily proportions that cause them to appear less flexible. Although there is an abundance of literature dealing with flexibility, a clear definitive statement regarding each of its many facets has not, as yet, been established. This is evidenced by a comprehensive review of the literature on the physiology of flexibility presented by Holland (1968). In addition to the different degrees of flexibility found among different persons, he indicates a consensus that there is a high degree of specificity of flexibility of the various joints of the body. The range of motion determined in one part of the body does not necessarily offer a predictive factor for flexibility in other body segments. Rasch and Burke (1967) also emphasize that flexibility is a specific factor for each joint.

Here again the SAID principle applies. As Holland (1968) reports, specific patterns of flexibility result from participation in physical activity that is specialized. With changes in range of motion coming about "naturally" by specialized forms of activity, it becomes evident that increased flexibility can be gained by adaptations to specifically imposed demands. This is done by regularly increasing effort while gradually increasing the demand for range of motion. Increased flexibility results from stretching the muscular membranes and tendons and by lengthening the ligaments and other tissues that limit the movement of the joint.

Two types of stretching procedures, one involving slow movements and the other rapid or ballistic motion, have been advocated by workers in this field. Studies regarding the value of both of these measures have been reported in recent years. Although Landreth (1957), who studied slow and fast stretching, and O'Connell (1960), investigating the relationship between static stretching and flexibility, found no significant changes, other more recent studies (de Vries, 1962; Logan and Egstrom, 1961) indicated significant improvement in the range of motion at the hip as a result of a training program

consisting of either slow or fast stretching procedures. A study by Hansen (1962) indicated that fast
or ballistic stretching with 15 repetitions of the performance of trunk flexion from the standing position produced significant increases in flexibility.

Most of these studies on the effects of slow and
fast stretching were performed over relatively short
periods of time and, therefore, yield limited information about the long-term effects of this type of
activity. However, there appears to be justification
for the preference of slow, controlled stretching procedures. In the studies of de Vries (1962) and Logan
and Egstrom (1961) muscle soreness was observed
by the subjects who performed the fast stretching
exercises. This has led de Vries (1962) to conclude
that slow or static stretching is recommended because it requires less expenditure of energy, will
probably result in less muscle soreness, and will
yield more qualitative relief from muscular distress.

As Holland (1968) has indicated, the myotatic
stretch reflex is one of the limiting physiological
factors to an increase of flexibility through various
methods of muscle stretching. When a muscle on
one side of a joint contracts and shortens, it is obvious that the muscle opposite the contracting muscle
must relax and lengthen. If relaxation in the muscle
opposite the action does not occur, movement would
not result. When stretching to increase flexibility, a
reflex inhibition occurs in the opposite or antagonistic muscle or muscle group (Loofbourrow, 1960).
It is hypothesized that reflex inhibition in the antagonistic muscle tends to lessen activated muscle
contraction caused by the stretch in that muscle and,
therefore, offers a greater potential for elongation
of the connective tissues involved.

The myotatic stretch reflex appears to be a
muscle protective mechanism and is apparently hy-
peractive in fast, uncontrolled stretching actions.
With the muscle resisting active stretch, the likeli-
hood of injury appears evident. Robert F. Shelton
(personal communication, 1949, University of Illinois) has suggested that this form of stretching used
prior to athletic events requiring violent bursts of
muscle contraction is a predisposing cause of sub-

sequent muscle injury. Ryan (1961) has emphasized that over-stretching muscles shortly before maximum stress may result in muscle tearing. Empirical observations of athletes tend to indicate that uncontrolled stretching of a ballistic nature may indeed increase the incidence of pulled or torn muscle tissue rather than decrease their incidence which is one of the original intents of the use of flexibility exercises in warm-up prior to performance. It seems feasible that actively contracting the muscles opposite those being stretched while moving through the range of motion in a slowly controlled manner offers the safest conditions for maximum lengthening of muscle tissue.

There is little scientifically determined evidence as to what constitutes an optimum level of flexibility for each individual. It has already been noted that flexibility is specific among individuals depending somewhat on the type of habitual activity. In addition, flexibility appears to be specific within different joints of the same person.

Extremes of flexibility are of little value in normal activity. The value of being reasonably flexible is the ability to move effectively and to maintain a relaxed, balanced body alignment. For this, normal joint motion is needed. Joint motion greater than normal may be either of use or a hindrance depending on whether sufficient strength is present to support the additional flexibility. For example, increased flexibility in the ankle joint might make it possible for the foot to have a greater range of motion and possibly result in the ability to exert more force in some movements. However, without the proper amount of strength and coordination to bear the weight of the body, the foot can be put in a very weak position. This, of course, can result in injury to the ankle. Less than normal flexibility, on the other hand, can cause injury as a result of inextensibility—the inability of the body part to "give."

The relationships between: (1) strength and flexibility and (2) strength development and subsequent changes in flexibility have been the concern of many investigators. A person can have the muscular system of his body highly developed in terms of strength and still be quite inadequate in physical activity. Though well equipped to handle the problems of strength, one might not be flexible enough to move easily and effectively. Connective tissues surrounding the muscle fibers are the structures mainly involved when muscles are being stretched. On the other hand, strengthening of muscle takes place largely in contractile muscle fibers. Therefore, strength and flexibility are for the most part independent of each other. However, it is possible to increase strength and at the same time increase or retain the flexibility of joints by purposefully applied flexibility exercises. It has long been a misconception that strength increases produce corresponding decreases in flexibility. A person exhibiting high strength levels has been termed *muscle-bound*. Claims that weight training causes a person to be "muscle-bound" and slow are groundless. One of the important early studies designed to test this belief was done by Massey and Chaudet (1956). They investigated the relationship between the use of systematic heavy resistance exercises on range of joint motion. An experimental group trained with weights for approximately six months during which time a control group participated in general physical education activities. Results indicated that weight training did not restrict bodily movements throughout the joints studied, with the exception of arm extension backward in an anterior—posterior plane from a position with the arms at the side of the body. Knee flexion increased but this was believed due to a forced knee flexion exercise. Later, Gardner (1963) studied the effects of both maximum isotonic or traditional weight training exercises and maximum isometric or static strength developing exercises and found no significant change in flexibility after a six-week training program. Other studies of a similar nature and empirical observations tend to corroborate Gardner's findings (Morehouse and Rasch, 1963).

Although scientific investigations tend to indicate little relationship between poor postural alignment and range of motion (Holland, 1968), clinical workers are of the opinion that habitual use of the flexor apparatus and weakened musculature resulting from inactivity may cause adaptive shortening of connective tissue. Since many of the studies of flexibility are performed using young subjects, the adaptive shortening seen in inactive older people with poor posture may not be evident at earlier ages. The often-seen imbalance of muscular strength on opposite sides of the joint seems to offer predisposing conditions for the occurrence of adaptive shortening of the connective tissue.

Some tissues, even though they are not contractile, serve an antigravity function. These include fascia in many parts of the body, especially the neck and lumbar regions. Any faulty postural situation in which the body is habitually held erect by fascia may cause adaptive shortening of these tissues. Because of the adaptive shortening that takes place as a result of the continual use or overuse of the flexor apparatus, inactive persons have a great need for flexibility. Compensation must be made for weakened muscles or faulty alignment in order for the body to be held upright against gravity. The shortened fascia and connective tissue take over the function of the weakened muscles. Thus the function of fascia may become over-efficient. If the fascia adapts to a shortened position the muscles on the opposite side of the joint may not be allowed to shorten completely when they contract. This prevents action through a full range of motion. A principal concern in flexibility development is to assure the development of the areas that have adaptively-shortened connective tissue due to weakened muscles on the opposite side.

A degree of caution should be observed when flexibility exercises are performed. The movements should be done slowly and without "bouncing" motions. Although the intensity with which one should stretch is difficult to ascertain, the movement should be to the point of pain and slightly beyond. Development of flexibility is a slow process. More intensity is required to increase the range of motion than to maintain it.

The role that is played by increasing the temperature of the tissues before performing flexibility exercises is not clear. Limited objective evidence is available regarding the relationship between these two variables. However, it is generally believed that increasing bodily temperature through exercises that elevate the cardiorespiratory function tends to increase the pliability of connective tissue, thus providing a greater potential for increased flexibility. Further, it is felt that the possibility of injury during the stretching period is lessened due to this generally elevated temperature in the body. In other words, exercises which are used for the development of endurance should precede stretching exercises in a general conditioning program.

The maintenance of adequate flexibility appears to depend upon the amount and intensity of movement of the body parts through complete ranges of motion several times a day. Since flexibility is an individual matter, each person must analyze his requirements for range of motion. As a safeguard against possible losses in flexibility, it is advisable to employ daily stretching exercises in each of those bodily areas commonly rendered inflexible by sedentary living. Flexibility exercises should also be performed prior to any strength training session.

II. FLEXIBILITY EXERCISES

Flexibility is best accomplished by slowly stretching until there is some discomfort—then stretching a bit further. While developing flexibility it is further recommended that the muscle opposite those being stretched be actively contracted during the exercise. For example, in an exercise in which the back of the thigh is stretched as the person is bending forward, a slow, sustained contraction of the abdominal and other anterior muscles is preferred to rapid, bouncing, stretching motions. Exercises for general body stretching are illustrated and described in the following section.

Stretch 1 (Figures 3.1, 3.2)
This hamstring stretch (Billig) is designed to increase the range of flexion in the lower back and at the hip joint. The arms are placed in the indicated position merely for convenience and balance. The

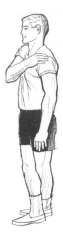

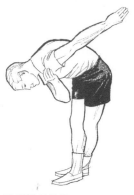

FIGURE 3.1
Billig Stretch, starting
position.

FIGURE 3.2
Billig Stretch, forward flex
position.

left leg is held as straight as possible, as the right
leg is placed in front of it (Figure 3.1). As one bends
slowly, contracting the abdominal muscles, the right
elbow is projected diagonally downward about five
times (Figure 3.2). This exercise should be repeated
to the opposite side.

Kinesiological Analysis:
Area most involved: lumbar spine, posterior hip, and
thigh.

Stretch 2 (Figures 3.3, 3.4)
The purpose of this exercise is to increase the range
of flexion in the lower back and at the hip joints.

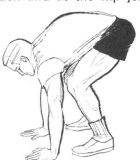

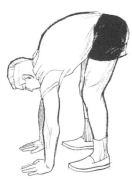

FIGURE 3.3   Hip and
Back Flexion Stretch,
starting position.

FIGURE 3.4   Hip and
Back Flexion Stretch.

The flexed hip and knee position is assumed first (Figure 3.3). Then an attempt is made to straighten the legs while the original position of the arms is maintained (Figure 3.4). The abdominal muscles should be strongly contracted as the legs are straightened.

Kinesiological Analysis:
Area most involved: lumbar spine, posterior hip, and thigh.

Stretch 3 (Figure 3.5)
This stretch is primarily designed to increase the range of flexion of the upper spine. The hands should be pressed downward against the floor and the abdominal muscles should be strongly contracted to facilitate the stretch.

Kinesiological Analysis:
Area most involved: thoracic and cervical spine.

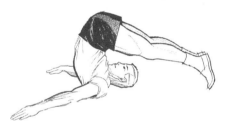

FIGURE 3.5   Upper Spine Stretch.

Stretch 4 (Figure 3.6)
This stretch is designed to increase the rotational flexibility of the spine. Facing forward, an attempt is made to twist the trunk as far as possible.

Kinesiological Analysis:
Area most involved: cervical, thoracic, and lumbar spine.

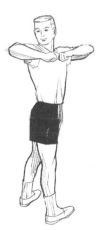

FIGURE 3.6   Spinal Rotation Stretch.

CHAPTER 3   References

de Vries, H. A. (1962). "Evaluation of Static Stretching Procedures for Improvement of Flexibility." *Research Quarterly of the American Association for Health, Physical Education, and Recreation* **33**:222–229.

Gardner, G. W. (1963). "Flexibility Changes as a Result of Isometric and Isotonic Exercise over a Limited Range of Motion." Unpublished doctoral Dissertation. University of Southern California, Los Angeles, California.

Hansen, T. O. (1962). "Selected Effects of Stretching on Flexibility." Unpublished master's thesis. University of California, Los Angeles, California.

Holland, G. J. (1968). "The Physiology of Flexibility: A Review." *In Kinesiology Review 1968*, pp. 49–62. American Association for Health, Physical Education, and Recreation, Washington, D.C.

Landreth, W. G. (1957). "A Comparative Study of Two Methods for Improving Range of Movement." Unpublished master's thesis. University of California, Los Angeles, California.

Logan, G. A., and Egstrom, G. H. (1961). "Effects of Slow and Fast Stretching on the Sacro-Femoral Angle." *Journal of the Association for Physical and Mental Rehabilitation* **15**(3):85–89.

Loofbourrow, G. N. (1960). "Neuromuscular Integration." *In Science and Medicine of Exercise and Sports* (W. R. Johnson, ed.), pp. 80–107. Harper, New York.

Massey, B. H., and Chaudet, N. L. (1956). "Effect of Systematic Heavy Resistance Exercise on Range of Joint Movement in Young Adults." *Research Quarterly of the American Association for Health, Physical Education, and Recreation* **27**:41–51.

Morehouse, L. E., and Rasch, P. J. (1963). *Sports Medicine for Trainers*. Saunders, Philadelphia, Pennsylvania.

O'Connell, E. G. (1960). "The Effect of Slow Stretching on Flexibility," Unpublished report. University of California, Los Angeles, California.

Rasch, P. J., and Burke, R. K. (1967). *Kinesiology and Applied Anatomy.* Lea & Febiger, Philadelphia, Pennsylvania.

Ryan, A. J. (1961). "The Role of Training and Conditioning in the Prevention of Athletic Injuries." *In Health and Fitness in the Modern World,* pp. 302–307. Athletic Institute, Chicago, Illinois.

FOUR/
Strength

FOUR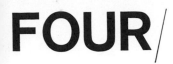

Muscle size and muscle strength are related. Throughout history references are made to the size, strength, and abilities of warriors and sportsmen. Men have known for thousands of years that hard work and vigorous training increases strength and hypertrophies muscle. But it is only recently that scientific investigations have helped to clarify the intensity and type of exercise stresses which develop and maintain muscular strength most efficiently.

Of all the physiological effects derived from participation in muscular activity, strength is undoubtedly one of the most essential (Clarke, 1960). For example, lack of strength is often a primary limiting factor when an attempt is made to improve skill. Although there is an interrelatedness among the physical fitness factors of strength, endurance, flexibility, and skill, without sufficient strength as a prerequisite, optimum levels of development of the other three factors will be greatly curtailed. In reviewing the values of exercise, particularly strength development, it becomes evident that it is the muscular system and the demands upon it that pull along the development of physical fitness in all the other systems of the body.

Physical fitness involves more than strength development. Too often programs of conditioning activities concentrate solely on the development of strength. Obviously these programs are shortsighted. Yet strength is an important prerequisite to other conditioning factors, and therefore, its advantages *and* limitations should be well understood in order for greatest benefits to be derived.

The amount of strength gain to be expected by the individual depends partly upon the level of his strength at the outset of the program. Those who have no previous participation in a strength development program can expect rather large increases while, on the other hand, persons with high-level strength at the beginning can expect very small increases. Then, too, due to the genetic make-up of the individual, some will tend to gain out of proportion to others. The ability to gain strength is related to individual differences just as is the acquisition of other abilities such as skill. Even though these differences do exist, diligently applied effort according to the methods suggested will provide significant gains.

The rate at which strength increases also varies among individuals. Generally, significant gains in strength can be noted after three or four weeks of training five periods per week for the beginner. In other words, 15 to 20 exercise periods will usually produce noticeable gains. Beyond that point gains will tend to accrue less dramatically and eventually level off with relatively smaller increases evidenced weekly.

Of all the components of physical fitness, more recent scientific investigations have been made about strength development and measurement than any others. A primary reason for the large volume of literature on this fitness factor relates not only to its importance to the organism but also to its complexity. Many of the studies have dealt with how strength is most effectively and efficiently developed. These studies have provided a sufficient basis upon which to formulate effective strength training programs. An understanding of the internal physiological adaptations is increasing. Some of the chemical and neurological changes which take place at the cellular level are known but others are yet to be elucidated.

I. MUSCLE FUNCTION AND TESTING

The function of a muscle is to develop tension within itself, thus showing a tendency to exert equal force on its two ends and pull them together toward the center. A muscle is not capable of pushing those ends apart. Therefore, muscles tend to be arranged in pairs on opposite sides of joints. One member of the pair is capable of bending the joint, the other member of straightening it. The members of the pair are said to be *antagonistic* to each other. The performing muscle is called the *agonist* (or muscle most involved) and the opposite muscle the *antagonist* (or contralateral muscle). In one joint action a muscle may be a muscle most involved; in another action that same muscle may be a contralateral muscle. This change depends upon the outside forces which come into play. Provided no outside forces enter the situation, pairs of muscles perform opposite functions. For example, the biceps brachii and brachialis muscles on the anterior surface of the arm are able to bend or flex the elbow joint. The triceps brachii muscle on the posterior surface of the arm is able to straighten or extend the elbow joint. Under certain circumstances, however, there is a modification of the concept of antagonistic action. Gravity, an outside force, may enter and modify the situation so that the arm can be first flexed and then extended while the biceps brachii and brachialis are tense and the triceps are relatively relaxed. Imagine a ten-pound weight held in the hand. If the biceps brachii and brachialis develop exactly ten pounds of effective tension, the weight may be held stationary. This is called *isometric* or static contraction. Although effort is being made and muscle tension is being developed, the lengths of the biceps brachii and brachialis remain unchanged. Next, if the muscles develop additional tension they will change their lengths, and the weight will be lifted as the elbow is flexed. This is called *concentric* or shortening contraction. Now suppose that the tension in the two muscles is reduced to less than ten pounds of effective tension. The force of gravity will overcome the tension in them and the arm will be straightened. In this case, gravity is responsible for moving the arm; the muscles act as a brake to prevent the elbow from snapping out of control as a result of the straightening action. As the elbow straightens the muscles will be lengthening, although they are still technically considered to be "contracted." Lengthening contraction is called *eccentric* contraction. In both concentric and eccentric contractions the body levers are moving. This type of contraction (wherein body levers move) is known as *isotonic* contraction. Strength development programs may involve increasing demands on the muscles either isometrically or isotonically.

Instruments for the measurement of strength have been in use for over 150 years. As early as 1807 Regnier of France is credited with designing the first practical spring dynamometer (Amar, 1920). His dynamometer was similar to the type of spring steel dynamometer which is used in strength testing today. Generally, strength measuring devices may employ the principle of metal deformation, spring balances, pneumatic systems, hydraulic devices, cable tensiometers, or electrical strain gauges (Hunsicker, 1955). These devices measure strength isometrically. Although Karpovich (1965) has reported the development of an isotonic strength measuring device, its introduction is too recent to have received widespread use. Practically all studies of strength development have used isometric measuring devices or have used data determined by the amount of weight which could be overcome by the subject isotonically through given ranges of motion. Individuals usually demonstrate greater efforts isometrically than isotonically. These differences are due to a greater number of factors operating in isotonic contractions than in isometric efforts. The factors include especially muscle length—force relationships, gravity, and changes in the angles of pull of the muscle and the angle of the joint. Further, isometric contractions permit greater stabilization of the involved joints, thus allowing more effort to be concentrated on the segment being measured and for the mobilization of more motor units within the muscle.

Figures 4.1–4.3 illustrate various methods for measuring strength. Whether strength is being measured by isometric or isotonic procedures, there is often a difference between true physiologic strength and the amount of strength which can be demonstrated at a particular time. This range between

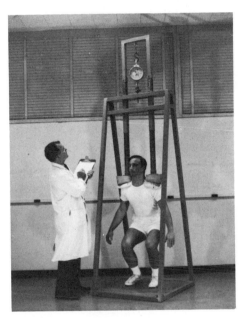

FIGURE 4.1
The Measurement of Leg Extension Strength. The subject uses the knee, hip, and ankle extensor muscles to supply force as he pushes with his shoulders against the padded part of the apparatus. The force of the push is indicated on the dynamometer at the top of the apparatus (Photo courtesy of Physical Education Research Laboratory, San Fernando Valley California State College).

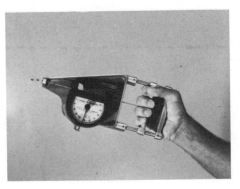

FIGURE 4.2
A Method for Measuring Grip Strength. By squeezing the hand grip, the individual exerts force through the short piece of aircraft cable. This force is recorded on the tensiometer (Photo courtesy of Physical Education Research Laboratory, San Fernando Valley California State College).

actually demonstrated ability and maximum capacity is dependent upon several factors. Lawther (1958) has stressed that an individual's ability to produce a maximum strength effort depends upon his motivation, background of punishing experience, and ability to withstand the pain of an all-out effort. Ikai and Steinhaus (1961) reported that performance of all-out maximal efforts are limited by psychological rather than physiological factors. Thus, the daily expression of strength may be highly variable. This variability must be taken into consideration when an assessment of the effectiveness of a training program is being made.

Although more force can be demonstrated isometrically than isotonically, this form of strength training may be less appealing than others. An advantage of isotonic exercise programs is the satisfaction of overcoming fixed amounts of resistance; it is possible to see what is accomplished. Effort does not

FIGURE 4.3
Recording the Right Knee Extension Strength by Using a Quadrant Assembly and Electronic Recorder. When the subject attempts the knee extension, a force is exerted through the aircraft cable on the front of the apparatus. The strain gauge dynamometer transmits the force to the recorder (rear) which records a force curve on the strip chart (Photo courtesy of Physical Education Research Laboratory, San Fernando Valley California State College).

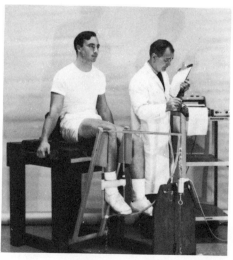

result in observable work in isometric exercise, although maximum exertions are made. Other differences between these two forms of exercise necessitate a more thorough understanding to guide intelligent application of each in a strength training program.

II. ISOMETRIC STRENGTH

The development of strength by isometric methods has received widespread attention in recent years. This is due largely to the fact that strength is gained without bodily movement, and therefore, the casual observer has assumed that no effort is required to perform such exercises. Although it is true that less time is needed to gain strength comparable to the gains derived from isotonic exercise, certain limitations of isometric exercise exist.

For many years isometric exercise was popularized as the Charles Atlas "dynamic tension" program. It was not until 1953 that much serious scientific attention was given to this form of exercise. At that time Hettinger and Müller (1953) of Germany reported their studies and observations on isometric exercise. Their method utilized static contractions applied at two-thirds maximal effort and held for six seconds. They reported that no further effort was required to yield gains of approximately five percent per week above the beginning level. Subsequent investigations in this country failed to yield such dramatic increases. Crakes (1957) duplicated the Hettinger–Müller technique and found only a two percent gain. Additionally, later studies by Müller and Rohmert, reported by Royce (1964), showed lower weekly increases than the original studies. Furthermore, the later studies utilized maximal contractions with as much as five seconds effort. Recent investigations (Ball et al., 1964; Rasch and Pierson, 1963; Rich et al., 1964) have employed maximum efforts with varying amounts of time and have demonstrated significant gains in strength. On the basis of these and similar investigations, it appears that one maximal contraction held for ten seconds is sufficient for maximum strength development in iso-metric training programs.

Although it has been demonstrated that significant isometric strength gains result from isometric train-ing, whether this increased strength can increase the force of isotonic contractions used in sports perform-ance and thereby improve the ability to perform, has not been sufficiently demonstrated. Many studies (Berger, 1963; Wolbers and Sills, 1956; Newlin, 1959; and Ball et al., 1964) indicate that although significant strength increases were found, the in-creased strength was not accompanied by an im-provement in a variety of isotonic skills. Furthermore, there appears to be little increase in muscular endurance subsequent to an isometric training program. Wells (1966) and Morehouse and Rasch (1963) indicate that cardiovascular endurance does not increase and that isometric exercise contributes only to the strength aspect of physical fitness.

It has long been held by physiologists that the amount of force that a muscle could exert was directly proportional to its anatomic cross section. The determination of this finding came from obser-vations made on electrically stimulated excised muscle to which known weights were attached. How-ever, measurements of volitional efforts of intact muscle, particularly after a training program with isometric exercise, do not necessarily yield compar-able results. Although gains in strength from isotonic exercise are generally proportional to an increase in the cross section of the muscle, Brouha (1962) has reported that gains in power may be three or more times greater than gains in muscle hypertrophy or girth.

Differences in hypertrophy between isometric and isotonic exercise may be due to less circulatory func-tion being required to perform isometric exercise. Since isometric exercise usually provides little gain in cardiorespiratory endurance it may be deduced that the increased capillarization does not occur. Morehouse and Miller (1963) believe that an in-creased number of capillaries supplying the muscle may account for increases in the hypertrophy which is usually demonstrated in isotonic exercise. Isometric exercise may, therefore, be of special value to the person desiring an increase in muscle strength or tone without a corresponding increase in hypertrophy.

One aspect of isometric exercise that may hold some promise for future investigations is the reduction of dimensions in specified areas of the body. Although the evidence is limited, Mohr (1965) claimed not only a reduction in the girth at the waistline and umbilical level of the abdomen in a group of adult women subjects, but also a significant reduction of subcutaneous fat. Similar findings were reported by Vandine (1964) who studied the girth of the hip and thigh muscles. These two studies indicate the possible efficiency of isometric exercise as a "spot reducer," but more study is required to validate this hypothesis. An earlier study by Day (1957) dealing with only the reduction of the waistline of women by maximum isometric contraction reported significant decreases in the waistline after a training program of six weeks. She indicated the results tended to regress at about the rate they were gained.

Isometric exercise is a valuable *supplement* to other exercises because of its simplicity and rapid results. Often, too little time or equipment is available to perform isotonic weight training exercises. In this situation isometric exercises can provide a rapid and convenient way to obtain strength. It is often used as a "home" program for youth and adults as well.

III. ISOTONIC STRENGTH

The type of exercise that has been most widely applied in the development of high level strength has been isotonic exercise. Although isometric exercise has been recommended for a most efficient gain in muscular strength for the amount of time invested, there are distinct advantages to be gained through isotonic exercise, and it is preferred for general use (Hellebrandt, 1962; Morehouse and Rasch, 1963).

Scientific investigation of weight training procedures for the development of strength received their initial impetus from the work of DeLorme (1945). At first he proposed the use of 70 to 100 repetitions utilizing weights with the repetitions being performed in sets of ten each. Originally termed heavy resistance exercise, he subsequently changed the name of the system to progressive resistance exercise. Later, it was suggested that the original number of repetitions was too high and that 20 to 30 were sufficient for each exercise (DeLorme and Watkins, 1951). The DeLorme method consists of determining by trial and error the most weight that can be lifted for ten repetitions. This is then called 10 R.M., or ten repetitions maximum. The exercises are then performed in sets or bouts of ten repetitions each. The first bout is with one-half the 10 R.M.; the second bout with three-fourths 10 R.M.; and the last bout with the 10 R.M. Most isotonic strength development programs currently in use employ this procedure or some modification of progressive resistance exercise. In general, modifications are in the total number of repetitions which are performed. Berger (1962), studying variations of resistances and repetitions, reported that six repetitions for three bouts yielded the greatest strength gains. Other investigations, when summarized, indicate that the use of one bout of five to fifteen repetitions performed with *maximum effort* is sufficient for each exercise period. A greater number of repetitions fail to yield significantly greater gains.

Muscle responds to imposed demands of a strength training program by increasing its endurance or ability to sustain effort as well as increasing strength and hypertrophy. This type of endurance is localized in the muscles which perform the exercise. Although circulatory increases may account for some of the increased muscular endurance, neurological adaptations are probably responsible for most of these changes. There appears to be a difference between localized muscular endurance and general cardiorespiratory endurance, which improves the over-all efficiency of the blood vascular system.

Isotonic strength gains have been found to be most markedly increased at the point in the range of motion where the greatest resistance is met

(Logan, 1960). This suggests that muscular endurance and strength may be a form of skill developed through training the neurological mechanism to make specific adaptations at given points in the range of movement. The muscle may have strength and endurance to perform one task but tasks of a different nature may be more difficult than would be anticipated. Again, this is substantiation for the SAID principle.

IV. STRENGTH—ENDURANCE RELATIONS

Strength and muscular endurance are interrelated. As emphasis is placed on one of these factors some ability to perform the other is gained. However, a certain minimum level of strength must be achieved before emphasis can be placed on endurance training. That is to say, strength appears to be prerequisite to muscular endurance. Lind and McNicol (1967) have shown that muscle tensions below 15 percent maximum voluntary contraction (MVC) can be held indefinitely without the onset of fatigue. At tensions above 15 percent MVC, blood flow is never sufficient to meet the metabolic requirements of the active muscles. The stronger a muscle is, the greater will be the absolute strength of a 15 percent MVC. Because of this fact, the stronger muscle will fatigue less readily during a given exercise.

Clarke (1960) has reported that the major factor leading to muscular strength improvement is the amount of tension developed in the muscle. Hellebrandt and Houtz (1956) have indicated that the critical variable in the improvement of strength and muscular endurance is the amount of work done per unit of time. The force—time relationship of strength and muscular endurance has led to the formulation of the concept of a strength—endurance continuum (Logan and Foreman, 1961). That such a continuum exists has been substantiated by Yessis (1963). A single maximal effort represents one end of the continuum while a maximum number of repetitions involving a constant resistance represents the other end of the continuum (See Figure 4.4). Points between these two extremes represent different ratios of resistances to repetitions. For example, when ten repetitions with maximum resistance for these repetitions are performed, strength and some endurance are gained. A point farther up the scale involving increased repetitions against a lesser fixed resistance will result in a greater gain in endurance and less gain in strength. Strength training methods consisting of combinations of repetitions and resistances which can be represented progressively along at least four points on this continuum are currently in use. The method to be used is dependent upon the ratio of strength to endurance desired. When training for a sport or other similar activity, the emphasis on strength or endurance or both will depend upon which of these is most important to the event.

V. CIRCUIT TRAINING

Yessis (1963) has shown that when approximately two-thirds of a maximum number of repetitions are performed against a fixed resistance, both strength and muscular endurance tend to be developed at an optimum rate for most purposes. This procedure, introduced as Circuit Training in England by Morgan and Adamson (1961) is a form of interval training for increasing strength and endurance with the individual doing increasing work in a given amount of

FIGURE 4.4
The Strength–Endurance Continuum. Low numbers of repetitions with heavy weight makes a proportionately greater contribution to strength than it does to endurance. Conversely, high numbers of repetitions with light weight makes a proportionately greater contribution to endurance. Both strength and endurance can be developed by choosing intermediate repetitions and weights.

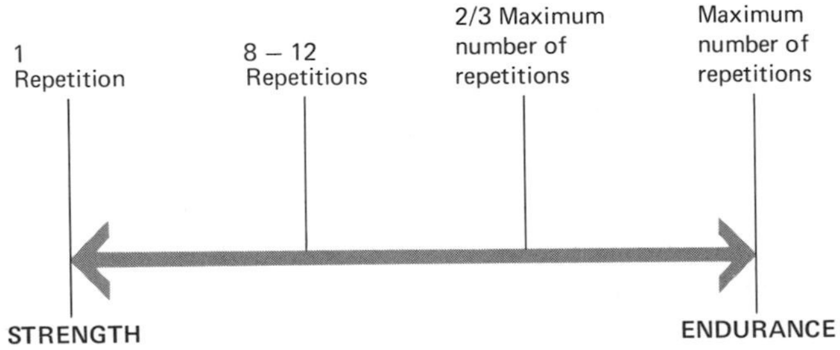

| 1 Repetition | 8 – 12 Repetitions | 2/3 Maximum number of repetitions | Maximum number of repetitions |

STRENGTH   ENDURANCE

time or the same work in a shorter period of time (Adamson, 1959). Several modifications of Circuit Training have been made in recent years. The most frequently used procedure involves a sequence of six to ten exercises that impose resistances that are arbitrarily established. At the outset of the training program, an effort is made to achieve a maximum number of repetitions for each exercise. Once this has been done, this maximum number is reduced by one-third for each exercise. The object is then to complete a circuit of all the exercises in a progressively diminishing amount of time. Early in the training program, for example, a circuit composed of 10 exercises may be completed three times in 30 minutes. This, of course, depends upon the number of exercises selected and the level of condition of the participants. To increase the demands, this procedure is intensified periodically by increasing the number of repetitions and the amount of resistance appropriately.

The following is an example of how a single exercise is employed in a circuit training program. If an exercise for elbow flexion such as biceps curls is included in the circuit, and 55 pounds of resistance has been arbitrarily established, and the person can perform 21 repetitions, the number of repetitions is decreased to 14 and the exercise is performed three times during the exercise period. That is, once during each circuit 14 repetitions of the biceps curl are performed. To intensify this exercise in the circuit, the number of repetitions and the amount of resistance are increased periodically. Although any group of exercises may be included in a circuit, a sequence of eight essential exercises purposely arranged in order to allow for distributed effort of body segments and an all-round body development are recommended, illustrated, and described in the next chapter.

VI. REPROPORTIONING

Strength development procedures offer a way of reproportioning the body. In general, unwanted adipose tissue can only be removed through a decrease in the number of calories consumed in the daily diet in contrast to what is needed to meet energy requirements. This unwanted fat may also be lost by increasing energy expenditure in contrast to calories consumed. A combination of these seems the most desirable. It has been observed that weight reduction programs first affect those areas of the body in which the fat was last deposited. Further, there appear to be variations from person to person in the distribution of fat deposits. Because of this, similar results cannot be expected in all individuals. Reproportioning can be effected not by moving fat from one location to another but by the development of muscular hypertrophy in some areas where recontouring is desired. Also, by increasing the tone of the muscles in such areas as the waistline, a greater ability to "hold in" the viscera is attained with an accompanying better appearance.

VII. STRENGTH AND AGE

One's greatest muscular strength is attained between the years of 20 and 30 (See Figure 4.5). Shock (1962) has indicated that a loss of bodily function over the years is related directly to loss of tissue and more particularly, to a disappearance of cells from muscles, the nervous system, and many vital organs. He reports, however, that little decline is seen in the nerves that connect to the muscles as a result of age. This factor may account for the fact that skill once attained is usually retained throughout one's lifetime. Steinhaus (1955) believes that

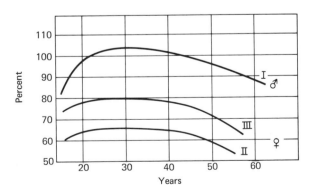

FIGURE 4.5
Isometric Strength in Relation to Age. Average of 25 different muscle groups. I, men; II, women; III, women corrected for size under the assumption that strength is proportional to $(height)^2$. The strength of 22-year-old men is used as a standard (equal to 100 percent) (From Asmussen, 1968).

strength maintained over a long period of time tends to become "anchored" in the muscle. DeLorme and Watkins (1951) have stated that muscle strength in later years is a reflection of former activity and that strength developed by strenuous activity is maintained indefinitely. The retention of the element of skill associated with strength appears to be a valid justification for early initiation and continuous participation in strength developing activities. Research by Asmussen and Mathiasen (1962) has indicated that individuals who continue physical activity into middle age show less of the strength decrease associated with aging shown in Figure 4.5.

CHAPTER 4   References

Adamson, G. T. (1959). "Circuit Training." *Ergonomics* **2**:183–186.

Amar, J. (1920). *The Human Motor*. Dutton, New York.

Asmussen, E. (1968). "The Neuromuscular System and Exercise." *In Exercise Physiology* (H. B. Falls, ed.), pp. 3–42. Academic Press, New York.

Asmussen, E., and Mathiasen, P. (1962). "Some Physiologic Functions in Physical Education Students Re-Investigated After Twenty-five Years." *J. Am. Geriat. Soc.* **10**:379–387.

Ball, J. R., Rich, G. Q., and Wallis, E. L. (1964). "Effects of Isometric Training on Vertical Jumping." *Research Quarterly of the American Association for Health, Physical Education, and Recreation* **35**:231–235.

Berger, R. A. (1962). "Effect of Varied Weight Training Programs on Strength." *Research Quarterly of the American Association for Health, Physical Education, and Recreation* **33**:168–181.

Berger, R. A. (1963). "Comparison between Static Training and Various Dynamic Training Programs." *Research Quarterly of the American Association for Health, Physical Education, and Recreation* **34**:131–135.

Brouha, L. (1962). "Physiology of Training, Including Age and Sex Differences." *Journal of Sports Medicine and Physical Fitness* **2**:3–11.

Clarke, H. H. (1960). "Development of Volitional Muscle Strength as Related to Fitness." *In Exercise and Fitness*, pp. 200–213. Athletic Institute, Chicago, Illinois.

Crakes, J. G. (1957). "An Analysis of Some Aspects of an Exercise and Training Program Developed by Hettinger and Muller." Unpublished master's thesis. University of Oregon, Eugene, Oregon.

Day, I. J. (1957). "A Study of the Reduction of the Waistline of Women by Maximum Isometric Contraction of the Abdominal Wall." Unpublished master's thesis. Louisiana State University, Baton Rouge, Louisiana.

DeLorme, T. L. (1945). "Restoration of Muscle Power by Heavy-Resistance Exercises." *Journal Bone Joint Surgery* **37A**:645–667.

DeLorme, T. L., and Watkins, A. L. (1951). *Progressive Resistance Exercise*. Appleton, New York.

Hellebrandt, F. A. (1962). "The Scientific Basis of Weight Training." *In Weight Training in Sports and Physical Education*. American Association for Health, Physical Education, and Recreation, Washington, D. C.

Hellebrandt, F. A., and Houtz, S. J. (1956). "Mechanisms of Muscle Training in Man: Experimental Demonstrations of the Overload Principle." *Physical Therapy Review* **35**:371–383.

Hettinger, T. and Müller, E. A. (1953). "Muskelleistung and Muskeltraining," *Internationale Zeitschrift fuer Angewandte Physiologie* **15**:111–125.

Hunsicker, P. A. (1955). "Arm Strength at Selected Degrees of Elbow Flexion." Technical Report 54–548, Project Number 7214. Wright Air Development Center, Wright-Patterson Air Force Base, Ohio.

Ikai, M. and Steinhaus, A. H. (1961). "Some Factors Modifying the Expression of Human Strength." *In Health and Fitness in the Modern World*, pp. 148–161. Athletic Institute, Chicago, Illinois.

Karpovich, P. V. (1965). *Physiology of Muscular Activity*. Saunders, Philadelphia, Pennsylvania.

Lawther, J. D. (1958). "The Pennsylvania State University Studies on Strength Development, Maintenance, and Related Aspects." *In Annual Proceedings, College Physical Education Association*, pp. 142–149. College Physical Education Association, Washington, D. C.

Lind, A. R., and McNicol, G. W. (1967). "Muscular Factors Which Determine the Cardiovascular Responses to Sustained and Rhythmic Exercise." *Canadian Medical Association Journal* **96**:706–713.

Logan, G. A. (1960). "Differential Applications of Resistance and Resulting Strength Measured at Varying Degrees of Knee Extension." Unpublished doctoral dissertation. University of Southern California, Los Angeles, California.

Logan, G. A., and Foreman, K. E. (1961). "Strength–Endurance Continuum" *The Physical Educator* **18**: 103.

Mohr, D. R. (1965). "Changes in Waistline and Abdominal Girth and Subcutaneous Fat Following Isometric Exercises." *Research Quarterly of the American Association for Health, Physical Education, and Recreation* **36**:168–173.

Morehouse, L. E., and Miller, A. T. (1963). *Physiology of Exercise*. Mosby, St. Louis, Missouri.

Morehouse, L. E., and Rasch, P. J. (1963). *Sports Medicine for Trainers*. Saunders, Philadelphia, Pennsylvania.

Morgan, R. E., and Adamson, G. T. (1961). *Circuit Training* Sportshelf & Soccer, New Rochelle, New York.

Newlin B. (1959). "The Relation of Isometric Strength Training to Isotonic Strength Performance." Unpublished master's thesis. University of California, Los Angeles, California.

Rasch, P. J., and Pierson, W. R. (1963). "Isometric Exercise, Isometric Strength, and Anthropometric Measurements." *Internationale Zeitschrift fuer Angewandte Physiologie* **20**:1–4.

Rich, G. Q., Ball, J. R., and Wallis, E. L. (1964). "Effects of Isometric Training on Strength and Transfer of Effect to Untrained Antagonists." *Journal of Sports, Medicine and Physical Fitness* **4**:217–220.

Royce, J. (1964). "Re-Evaluation of Isometric Training Methods and Results, A Must." *Research Quarterly of the American Association for Health, Physical Education, and Recreation* **35**:215–216.

Shock, N. W. (1962). "The Physiology of Aging." *Scientific American* **206**(1):100–110.

Steinhaus, A. H. (1955). "Strength from Morpurgo to Müller—A Half Century of Research." *Journal of the Association for Physical and Mental Rehabilitation* **9**:147–150.

Vandine, D. (1964). "A Comparison of the Effects of Isometric and Isotonic Exercises on Reduction of Girth of the Glutei and Thigh Muscles." Unpublished master's thesis. State University of Iowa, Iowa City, Iowa.

Wells, K. F. (1966). *Kinesiology*. Saunders, Philadelphia, Pennsylvania.

Wolbers, C. P., and Sills, F. D. (1956). "Development of Strength in High School Boys by Static Muscle Contractions." *Research Quarterly of the American Association for Health, Physical Education, and Recreation* **27**:446–450.

Yessis, M. (1963). "Relationships between Varying Combinations of Resistances and Repetitions in the Strength–Endurance Continuum." Unpublished doctorial dissertation. University of Southern California, Los Angeles, California.

FIVE/ Strength Training Procedures

FIVE/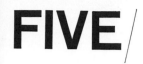

The most widely used form of exercise for the development of strength is isotonic or movement exercise. This form of exercise also develops cardiorespiratory and muscular endurance and increases the cross section of the muscle.

The isotonic conditioning exercises described in this chapter are designed to progressively apply resistance and develop a maximum of strength in a minimum of time. In general, these strength developing exercises involve the use of weights which are moved against the resistance of gravity. For individuals with lower tolerance for exercise, the body weight alone may serve as adequate resistance until the ability to overcome more resistance is gained. Wherever possible, barbells instead of dumbbells are recommended because of their adaptability and convenience.

Since the force of gravity remains constant regardless of the body position, it is often necessary to change the position of the body in order to apply resistance in a desired manner. In some exercises, equipment such as incline boards, leg press machines, or other apparatus provide for the position

FIGURE 5.1

Abdominal Area. Basic to any weight training program is the strengthening of the trunk muscles. In order to place the greatest stress on the abdominal muscles, the knees are flexed and the feet are held down by a strap on a slant board. By placing the knees in this position for the sit-up, less of the action is accomplished by the muscles which flex the hip. The abdominal muscles are required to perform more of the work.
Kinesiological Analysis. Muscles most involved: rectus abdominis, oblique externus abdominis, oblique internus abdominis, transversus abdominis.

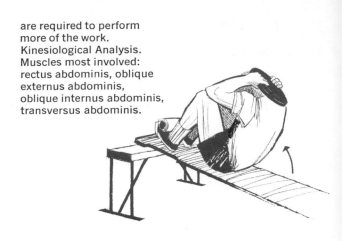

FIGURE 5.2

Posterior Trunk, Hip, and Thighs. (a) To strengthen the posterior trunk, hip, and thighs, the feet should be secured with a strap attached to a table. (b) The upper body should not be moved higher than parallel to the table in this trunk-raise exercise. A folded towel may be placed under the weight for added comfort.
Kinesiological Analysis. Muscles most involved: erector spinae, gluteus maximus, biceps femoris, semitendinosus, semimembranosus.

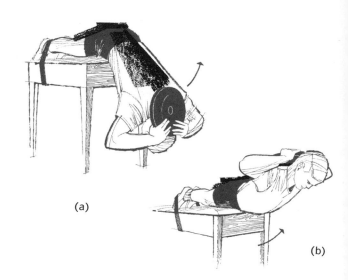

(a)

(b)

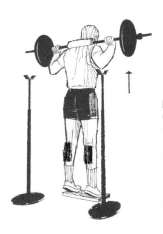

FIGURE 5.3

Calf Area. This calf-strengthening heel raise exercise involves the use of a raised surface (approximately two inches) to provide an increased range of motion for the ankle joint. Racks on which the barbell is placed prior to the exercise are essential when spotters are not available. A towel wrapped around the bar as illustrated prevents discomfort to the neck area.
Kinesiological Analysis. Muscles most involved: gastrocnemius, soleus.

changes which permit more effective application of resistance.

The speed and efficiency of strength development depends upon the number of repetitions, the amount of resistance, and other factors outlined below.

I. INTENSIFICATION OF IMPOSED DEMANDS

Progressively overcoming increased resistances is necessary for the development of strength. Studies concerning the optimum resistance and number of repetitions for the maximum gain in strength were discussed in the previous chapter. Although no precise resistance or number of repetitions has been advocated conclusively (Berger, 1962; Berger and Harris, 1966), it appears that for maximum strength gain no more than 12 or less than 6 repetitions need be performed for any one exercise. In order to determine the exact amount of resistance required to impose demands within this range, trial and error is required. One must experiment to find the amount of weight which allows the repetitions to remain within the range. If more than 12 repetitions can be

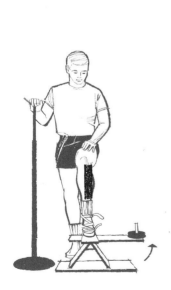

FIGURE 5.4
Ankle Area. This exercise is designed to strengthen the muscles of the ankle by the specific application of resistance to the muscles of the medial, lateral, and anterior aspects of the ankle. The device illustrated consists of a pivotable foot plate on a hinged lever arm to which weights can be attached. The weight rack simply provides a means of balance. The foot is secured to the foot plate of the ankle while the leg is held in the position shown. To exercise the anterior muscles, the foot plate is pivoted so that the weight is in the front of the foot. The movement should be a pulling action rather than a push with the heel. In order to exercise the medial muscles of the ankle, the plate is again pivoted, this time with the lever arm opposite that shown in the illustration. Care should be taken to avoid movement of the leg. Resistance should be increased so that no more than ten repetitions with maximum weight are possible. Kinesiological Analysis. Muscles most involved: Lateral aspect: peroneus longus, peroneus brevis, peroneus tertius; Anterior aspect: tibialis anterior, extensor digitorum longus, extensor hallucis longus, peroneus tertius; Medial aspect: tibialis anterior, tibialis posterior, flexor digitorum longus, flexor hallucis longus.

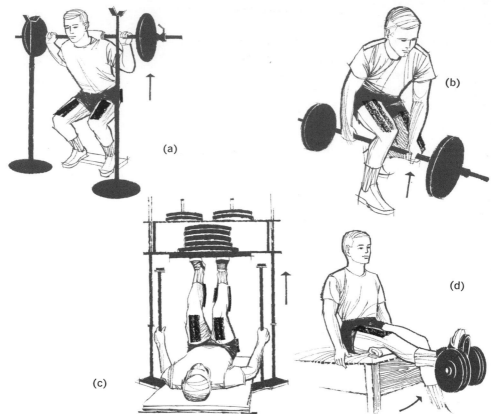

FIGURE 5.5
Hip, Ankle, Anterior Thigh. The illustrations in this figure show four approaches for use in strengthening the extensor muscles of the hip, knee, and ankle. In (a) a support is placed under the heels for stability and a towel is rolled on the bar for protection during the squat exercise. Before the exercise is begun, the barbell is placed on the supporting rack. The knees should not be bent beyond the position illustrated because of possible injury to the joint. (b) is an alternate method for strengthening the leg extensors. The knees should be completely extended and the weight lowered again to the floor. The back should be kept as straight as possible. (c) illustrates a leg press apparatus to which weights can be attached. This is the preferred method of developing strength in the leg and hip extensors. The device allows for a specific application of resistance to the extensor muscles of the hip, knee, and ankle joints in addition to offering maximum safety. In order to avoid extreme flexion of the knees as the weight is lowered, the knees should remain about the same distance apart throughout the exercise. In other words, the thighs should come in contact with the chest and not be allowed to spread apart. The position under the device should be such that when the thighs contact the chest the lower back and sacrum should remain in contact with the floor. (d) illustrates the use of an iron boot to which weights are attached. This knee extension exercise is used to concentrate the effort within the quadriceps femoris group of muscles. A folded towel is placed under the knee joint to promote comfort. Full extension of the knee should be obtained on each repetition.
Kinesiological Analysis. Muscles most involved: In (a), (b), and (c), gluteus maximus, biceps femoris, semitendinosus, semimembranosus, quadriceps femoris, gastrocnemius, soleus; In (d), quadriceps femoris.

performed with a given weight, the weight should be increased to bring the number of repetitions down to not less than 6. During each workout period an attempt should be made to increase the number of repetitions.

A few repetitions against a maximum resistance result in mostly strength while many repetitions against a lighter resistance result primarily in endurance. In both cases some of each is developed.

Experience has shown that when the tolerance for exercise has reached a very high level only small gains can be expected from an exercise period. Often no appreciable gains can be demonstrated. This is often referred to as a *plateau*. When this state is reached, it has been found that by attempting to lift heavier loads than can be handled may be effective in pushing one's tolerance to a higher level. For example, in the leg press exercise enough weight should be placed on the apparatus to allow the individual to almost perform one repetition. Several attempts should be made to overcome this resistance during the exercise period. This procedure should not be attempted more than once every week and is intended only as a supplement to the daily training procedure previously described.

Another method shown by experience to offer a way of overcoming a "plateau" is known as *cheating*. This consists of attempting to handle more weight than can be moved through a range of motion in the usually prescribed fashion for a given exercise. For example, in the biceps curl exercise, if the individual normally curls 50 pounds for 8 repetitions, he should increase the weight by approximately 20 percent or by 10 pounds and perform the exercise by using momentum resulting from "throwing" the trunk from a semi-flexed to an extended position. This is recommended only when an attempt is made to break the "plateau." This procedure is sometimes called a *power training program.*

II. REGULARITY

Exercise demands should be imposed at least three times a week and usually not more than five times

FIGURE 5.7
Arms and Chest. (a) shows the bench press exercise which is designed to strengthen the muscles of the arms and chest. Before one assumes the illustrated position, the barbell should be placed on the rack. Assistance may be required to place the weight in the exercise position as well as to remove it after ten repetitions against maximum resistance.
(b) is an alternative bench press utilizing an inclined board. This position allows greater emphasis to be placed on the upper chest and shoulder muscles.
(c) illustrates the use of dumbbells for chest and arm strength development. This exercise applies resistance specifically to the muscles of the chest. The weights should be raised and lowered through as great a range of motion as possible. It may be necessary to bend the elbows slightly to stabilize the elbow joint.

FIGURE 5.6
Posterior Thigh. This exercise applies resistance specifically for strength development in the knee flexors. A support is used to assure body balance. The exercise may be done while standing on a low bench to allow the foot to move through a greater range of motion.
Kinesiological Analysis. Muscles most involved: biceps femoris, semitendinosus, semimembranosus.

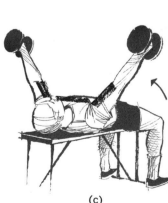

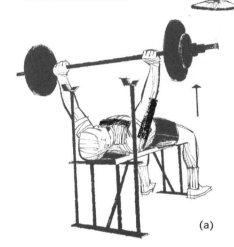

(a)

Kinesiological Analysis. Muscles most involved: In (a) and (b), triceps brachii, pectoralis major, pectoralis minor, coracobrachialis, short head of biceps brachii, anterior deltoideus, serratus anterior; In (c), pectoralis major, pectoralis minor, coracobrachialis, short head of biceps brachii, anterior deltoideus, serratus anterior.

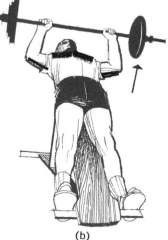

(b)

(c)

a week (Mathews and Kruse, 1957). However, in the highly motivated individual at the beginning stages of training, daily workouts may be desirable. As the condition of the person is improved, less frequent exercise periods may be required.

III. RANGE OF MOTION

Whenever appropriate, each exercise should be performed to the limit of joint action. Each movement should be forced as far as possible in order to promote flexibility of the joints. In some instances limiting the range of motion is recommended in order to protect other structures of joints. These exceptions are noted in the text. This is one reason for flexibility exercises to supplement isotonic conditioning. However, if incomplete movements are habitually performed, adaptive shortening of the connective tissues may occur.

IV. BREATHING

There is a tendency to hold the breath during extreme efforts to overcome heavy resistances. Holding the breath may have undesirable effects on the organism. When overcoming heavy resistances, the tendency to hold the breath creates a hazard. Under these conditions the abdominal muscles contract and the glottis closes. Pressures in the thoracic and abdominal areas are drastically increased by the breath being held. This inhibits the venous return of blood to the heart causing a fall in the blood pressure in the arteries. Arterial pressure decrease results in a reflex increased rate of the heart. After the effort of overcoming the heavy resistance, venous flow surges into the heart causing an increase in blood pressure in the pulmonary pathways. At this time, the systolic blood pressure may rise to over 200 millimeters of mercury (DeLorme and Watkins, 1951; Jones, 1965). This is known as the *Valsalva phenomenon*.

Although the Valsalva phenomenon may not be a hazard to the individual with a normal, healthy, circulatory apparatus, the possibility exists that medically undetected weaknesses in the system may be present. Therefore, in order to lessen the intensity of this potential hazard, it is recommended that the individual maintain an open glottis by breathing during the most difficult phase of the exercise. Also, by performing several repetitions with a lighter weight than could be lifted with one maximal effort, it is believed that the Valsalva phenomenon is less likely to result in injury.

It must be understood, however, that the way in which one breathes has nothing to do with the development of strength but that retaining an open glottis is employed only as a factor of safety.

V. MAINTENANCE OF STRENGTH

Once desired levels of strength are reached through a strength training program, the principle of progression need not apply. In order to maintain strength at a desired level, an increase in demand is not nec-

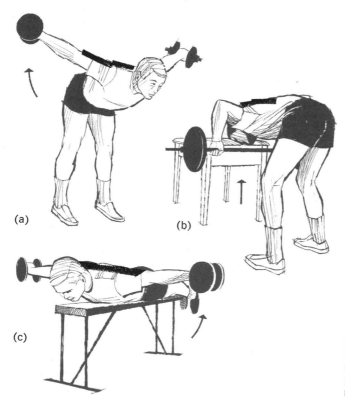

(a)

(b)

(c)

FIGURE 5.8   Upper Back. The main purpose of this exercise is to strengthen the muscles that hold the shoulder blades in proper alignment. This may be done in either the standing or lying positions shown. The trunk must be horizontal so that the pull of gravity is in the proper direction. Barbells or dumbbells may be used with equal effectiveness. The use of the table on which the forehead is placed provides stability in the standing position. Kinesiological Analysis. Muscles most involved: middle trapezius, rhomboideus major, rhomboideus minor, posterior deltoideus, teres major, triceps brachii.

essary. For the maintenance of strength a minimum
of two periods per week are recommended.

VI. SAFETY FACTORS

In addition to the procedure for preventing the Valsalva phenomenon, some other safety precautions
bear mentioning.

During the weight training routine, there is a
tendency for the palms of the hands to perspire.
Perspiration on the bars to which the weights are
attached can be counteracted with the use of chalk.
Chalk blocks in the form of carbonate of magnesia
can be purchased from gymnastic supply companies.

Since the equipment used in the weight training
program is detachable to allow for rapid changes of
the metal plates, caution must be taken to see that

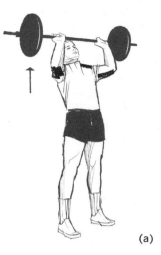

(a)

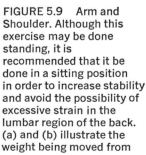

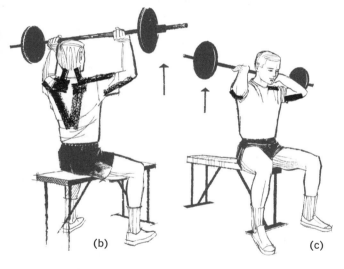

(b)   (c)

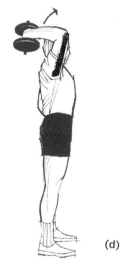

(d)

FIGURE 5.9   Arm and
Shoulder. Although this
exercise may be done
standing, it is
recommended that it be
done in a sitting position
in order to increase stability
and avoid the possibility of
excessive strain in the
lumbar region of the back.
(a) and (b) illustrate the
weight being moved from

the beginning chest level
position. With the weight
in front of the body, effort
is concentrated on the
anterior shoulder muscles.
(c) is an alternate position
with weight behind the
head. With this position
more emphasis is placed
on the extensors of the
elbow. (d) shows a
dumbbell being used to

apply resistance
specifically to the elbow
extensor muscles. The
upper arm should remain in
a vertical position during
the exercise.
Kinesiological Analysis.
Muscles most involved:
In (a), (b), and (c),
trapezius, serratus anterior,
deltoideus, triceps brachii;
In (d), triceps brachii.

the collars and other apparatus are securely attached. Further, it should be noted that metal plates
should never be placed on the ends of the bars without the use of collars. Most weight training injuries
result from insecurely attached equipment falling on
the feet and legs.

The beginner should not attempt to overcome
more resistance than can be safely handled. It is a
wise procedure to begin with about ten pounds less

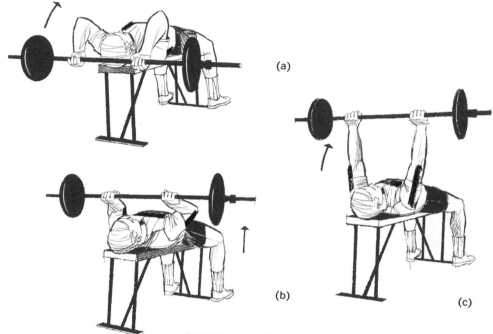

(a)

(b)

(c)

FIGURE 5.10   Chest and Arms. This figure illustrates three progressive stages of a pull-over exercise. It is recommended for the development of the latissimus dorsi muscle when only barbells are available. The exercise is begun with the arms bent. The angle of the elbows does not change until the upper arm is nearly vertical, at which time the elbow is straightened. Caution should be taken to avoid excessive resistance when beginning this exercise in order to minimize the possibility of injury to the shoulder joint. Kinesiological Analysis. Muscles most involved: latissimus dorsi, teres major, pectoralis major, pectoralis minor, rhomboideus major, rhomboideus minor, triceps brachii, coracobrachialis, short head of biceps brachii.

than one feels can be successfully overcome. Too often, injuries result from the inability to handle weight at the initiation of the program.

The use of spotters when performing such exercises as bench presses and squats is essential particularly when heavy loads are being managed. Racks to hold the weights preliminary to the exercise help eliminate some of the hazard involved.

One common fault in performing weight training exercises is attempting to lift weights from the floor while standing with the knees locked in a position of extension and the hips bent to approximately 90 degrees. The bent rowing exercise is a case in point. There has been much criticism of weight training because of back injuries resulting from improper positioning when this exercise is performed. If performed in a quick jerky fashion with the knees locked, severe damage can occur to the intervertebral discs of the spinal column. As the weight is lifted, undue pressure is placed on the intervertebral discs which forces the nucleus pulpsus, the fluid-like center of the disc, to project posteriorly. If the disc has any weakness due to previous injury or other causes, it may herniate and exert pressure on the spinal cord. This pressure results in a number of complications usually requiring medical attention (Keegan, 1953). Two ways of preventing this potential hazard are: (1) resting the forehead on a padded table while the lift is being performed, and (2) by bending the knees to about 15 degrees of flexion. These positions release the tension from the

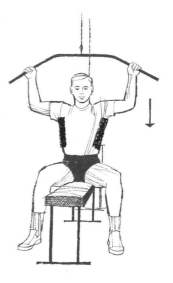

FIGURE 5.11
Chest and Arms. This illustration shows the use of a latissimus machine. Weights are attached by way of an overhead pulley. The exercise is begun with the elbows straight and completed with the bar either in back or in front, depending upon whether concentrated effort is desired in the upper back or the chest. In addition to the latissimus dorsi muscle, stress is placed as well on the elbow flexors rather than the extensors as in the pull-over of Figure 5.10. Kinesiological Analysis. Muscles most involved: latissimus dorsi, teres major, pectoralis major, pectoralis minor, rhomboideus major, rhomboideus minor, lower trapezius, coracobrachialis, biceps brachii, brachialis, brachioradialis.

posterior muscles of the thigh and back thereby allowing the lumbar spine to retain a normal curvature.

When lifting weights to move them from one place to another, the knees should be bent before the lift is made. This is sometimes called lifting from the number "4" position rather than from the number "7" position. These positions are so-named because the position the body assumes is similar to the numbers four or seven. When making such a lift, the legs and not the back should perform most of the action.

A thorough warm-up to elevate the body temperature and to provide an opportunity for stretching the muscles is essential preliminary to the strength training routine. The warm-up should consist of a series of total body movements designed to increase the circulatory function of the body. Exercises such as rapidly repeated jumps into the air from both feet, running in place, or rapidly repeated sit-ups are useful for the warm-up session. The rate of the exercise should be high enough so that the activity cannot be extended beyond one minute.

VII. STRENGTH DEVELOPMENT EXERCISES

Strength training exercises for the various muscle groups of the body are pictured throughout this chapter (Figures 5.1–5.18). Dark shaded areas of the body show the location of the muscles most involved. For each of the exercises, it is recommended that the number of repetitions with maximum resistance not exceed ten. If more than twelve repetitions

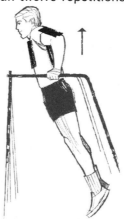

FIGURE 5.12   Chest and Arms. In this figure we see the use of parallel bars on which a dipping exercise is performed. With this exercise the elbow extensors receive much stress as well as the muscles of the chest. Kinesiological Analysis. Muscles most involved: latissimus dorsi, teres major, pectoralis major, pectoralis minor, rhomboideus major, rhomboideus minor, lower trapezius, triceps brachii, coracobrachialis, short head of biceps brachii.

can be performed, more resistance should be added. On the other hand, the resistance is too heavy if the movement cannot be done at least six times.

A description and kinesiological analysis of each exercise are given as part of the figure legends. Table 5.1 will give the student a basis for comparing himself with others of similar age and weight for a few of the exercises.

Table 5.1
Britten Achievement Standards*

Body Weight	Excellent†	Good†	Average†

Sit-up—See Figure 5.1
10-pound weight held behind head, knees flexed to 90 degree angle and feet held down.

135	45	25	10
155	50	30	15
175	55	35	20
195	60	40	25

Back Extensions—See Figure 5.2
Trunk extended over end of table, 10-pound weight held behind neck with both hands, head is lifted above level of table top each time.

135	75	30	10
155	85	40	15
175	95	50	25
195	105	60	35

Biceps Curl (barbell)—See Figure 5.13
55 pounds of weight, back against wall to prevent "cheating," bar touches thighs when down, elbows must be fully flexed when up. Heels must remain on floor and knees not bent.

135	70	50	40
155	80	60	50
175	90	70	60
195	100	80	70

Squats (125 pounds)—See Figure 5.5
Bar behind neck on pad, squat to point where thighs are horizontal.

135	210	135	110
155	220	150	120
175	235	165	135
195	250	175	150

* Data compiled by Sam D. Britten, San Fernando Valley State College. Based on measurements made 1960–1967 on lower division college men.
† Indicates number of repetitions to be done for each category.

VIII. CIRCUIT TRAINING

The origin and physiological foundations of circuit training were discussed in Chapter Four. They are based on the work of Adamson (1959) and Morgan and Adamson (1961). The operational phase of this type of program bears repeating here. The unique concept of circuit training is that exercise stress is applied within the capability of each individual performer. In brief, a sequence of exercises, the number depending upon the available time and the desired outcomes, is selected. If the available time is short, a series of five exercises are recommended as follows: sit-up, back extension, squat, overhead press, and biceps curl. The sequence is purposely

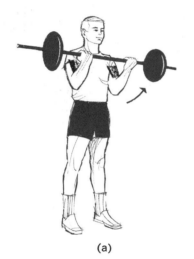

(a)

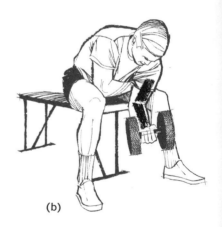

(b)

FIGURE 5.13   Arms. This exercise, the biceps curl, strengthens the flexor muscles of the elbow and wrist. The position with the palms up intensifies the action of the wrist flexors. If the weight were held with the palms down, greater stress would be placed on the extensors of the wrist. As far as strengthening the elbow flexors is concerned, there is little difference in the two hand positions. When concentration of effort on one arm is desired, the use of a dumbbell as shown in (b) is recommended. In both (a) and (b) care should be taken to avoid moving the trunk backward and thus swinging the weight up. Kinesiological Analysis. Muscles most involved: biceps brachii, brachialis, brachioradialis.

arranged in this order to avoid two consecutive exercises in the same general area of the body. These five exercises are basic to any conditioning program. The first three are specifically related to the development of the antigravity muscles discussed in Chapter One. They work on the extensor muscles at the ankle, knee, hip, and back and the flexors of the trunk—the abdominal muscles. The other two exercises are for the development of the chest and arms. Although the only exercises shown utilize weights, circuit training stations may involve other available equipment such as horizontal bars, parallel bars, horizontal ladders, and other gymnastic type apparatus.

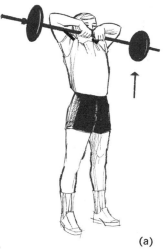

(a)

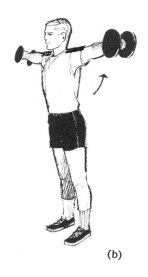

(b)

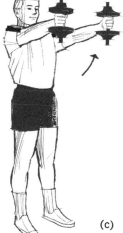

(c)

FIGURE 5.14   Shoulders. (a) illustrates the erect rowing exercise designed to place particular stress on the deltoideus muscles. The beginning position is with the weight held just below the waist. (b) pictures an alternate exercise using dumbbells to strengthen the deltoideus. The starting position here is with the weights held at the sides. In (c) a dumbbell exercise is shown that places most of the stress on the anterior portion of the deltoideus. The starting position is with the weights at the sides. Kinesiological Analysis. Muscles most involved: In (a), deltoideus, trapezius, serratus anterior, biceps brachii, brachialis, brachioradialis. In (b), deltoideus, trapezius, serratus anterior; In (c), anterior deltoideus, serratus anterior, upper pectoralis major, coracobrachialis, short head of biceps brachii.

FIGURE 5.15 Shoulder Girdle. The exercise shown here develops strength in the muscles that elevate the shoulder girdle.

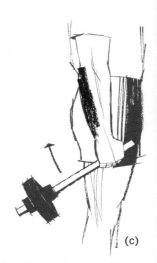

Kinesiological Analysis. Muscles most involved: upper trapezius, levator scapulae, rhomboideus major, rhomboideus minor.

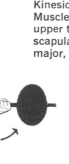

(a)

FIGURE 5.16.   Forearm. These drawings picture exercises which strengthen the muscles acting at the wrist joint. (a) shows an exercise which is utilized for both the wrist flexors and extensors. With the forearms resting on the thighs, the wrists are flexed and extended through a full range of motion. With the weight held in the palms up position, the wrist flexors are stressed. In the palms down position, the stress is placed on the extensors. (b) shows an exercise which is used to strengthen the muscles on the thumb side of the wrist. The weight should be raised and then lowered from the starting position without movement of the forearm. (c) shows the starting position for a

(b)

(c)

similar exercise that strengthens the muscles on the little finger side of the wrist.
Kinesiological Analysis. Muscles most involved: In (a) (Palms up position), flexor carpi radialis, flexor carpi ulnaris, flexor digitorum superficialis, flexor digitorum profundus;

(a) (Palms down position), extensor carpi radialis longus, extensor carpi radialis brevis, extensor digitorum, extensor carpi ulnaris; In (b) flexor carpi radialis, extensor carpi radialis longus, extensor carpi radialis brevis; In (c), flexor carpi ulnaris, extensor carpi ulnaris.

For all-round body development of both strength and muscular endurance the eight station circuit training program illustrated in Figure 5.19 is recommended. Each day, prior to utilization of this training program, a warm-up consisting of at least one cardiorespiratory activity from Chapter Seven and the four flexibility exercises in Chapter Three should be performed.

At the outset of the program, an effort should be made to achieve a maximum number of repetitions for each of the eight exercises. Once this has been recorded, the number is reduced for each exercise by approximately one-third. The objective then becomes the completion of the circuit through all the exercises in a progressively diminishing amount of time. Completing the circuit means doing, in sequence, all the exercises. During the circuit each exercise should be done in a minimum amount of time. The circuiut may then be repeated. That is, the exercises may be done in the same order a scond or third time. The amount of time it takes to complete the circuit, of course, depends upon the level of condition of the individuals participating. To impose increased demands, this procedure is altered periodically, usually every two to three weeks, by increasing the number of repetitions and, when appropriate, the amount of resistance applied.

As indicated in Chapter Four, the following is an example of how a single exercise is employed in a circuit training program: If an exercise for elbow flexion, such as biceps curls is to be performed, and 55 pounds of resistance has been arbitrarily estab-

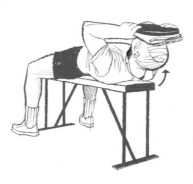

FIGURE 5.17   Neck. The purpose of this exercise is to develop the strength of the anterior neck muscles. The starting position is with the head hanging over the end of the bench. A folded towel on which the weight is placed is used for added comfort.
Kinesiological Analysis. Muscle most involved: sternocleidomastoideus.

lished for that station, and the person can perform 21 repetitions, the number of repetitions is decreased to 14 and the exercise is performed three times during the exercise period. That is, once during each circuit, 14 repetitions are performed with the biceps curl.

The arbitrary establishment at each of the stations should be guided by the general tolerance of the individuals participating. Experience has shown that the weight should be light enough to permit a low-tolerance individual to perform at least 10 repetitions and heavy enough for those of higher tolerance to perform not more than 30 repetitions during the initial repetition determination day. Often, because of a wide range of exercise tolerance among groups it becomes necessary to provide weights with different poundages at the various stations. For example, at the squat station, which usually requires more time to complete than the others, fixed barbells of 100 and 125 pounds may be provided. Once

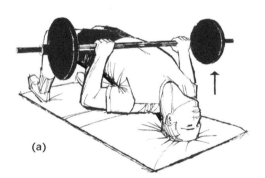

(a)

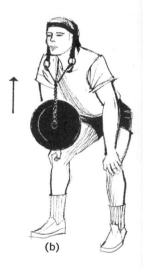

(b)

FIGURE 5.18   Posterior Hip and Spine. (a) shows an exercise which develops the strength of the extensor muscles of the hip and back, with particular stress placed on the neck extensors. It should be performed on a padded surface. With the barbell in place on the chest, movement is made from a lying position with the knees and hips flexed.

(b) shows an exercise which is designed to localize the stress in the posterior neck area. The head should be moved upward and downward with a weight atttached to a head harness.
Kinesiological Analysis. Muscles most involved: In (a), erector spinae, gluteus maximus; In (b), upper portion of erector spinae, upper trapezius.

the weights have been adjusted for the tolerance range of the group, they should not be increased for at least two to three weeks.

Early in the training program, a circuit composed of eight exercises may be completed three times in approximately 25 minutes. Since circuit training has particular application to school programs and large numbers of individuals may be participating in one circuit, it has been found that there is a tendency for the performance of the circuit to be slowed because of the time required for certain of the exercises. In order to facilitate the exercise procedure at these slower stations, it is often desirable to have two sets of weights available. Furthermore, if for example, 24 individuals were involved with the circuit at one time, they might well work in groups of three each and remain in these groups as they move from station to station. This is particularly advantageous from the standpoint of assistance in the handling of the weights, spotting, and other safety procedures.

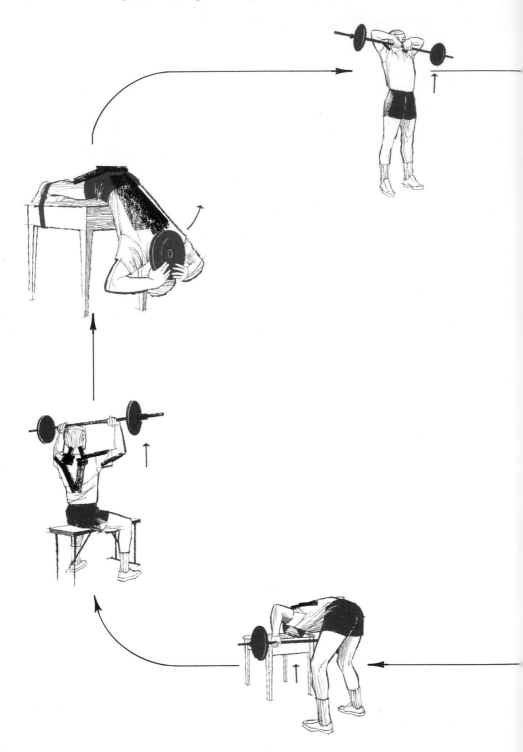

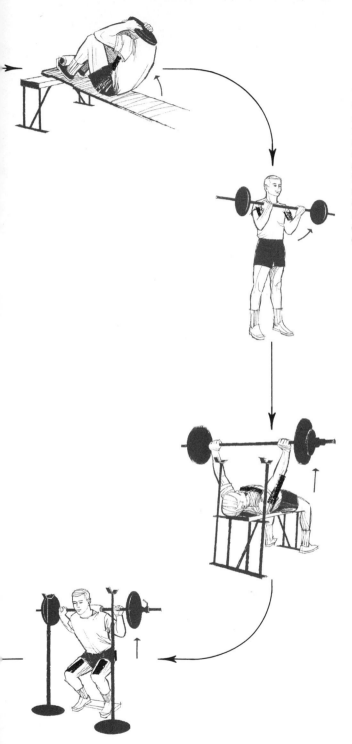

FIGURE 5.19
Recommended Circuit Training Stations. Circuit training application of these eight stations will train all the large muscle groups of the body. The circuit should be followed in clockwise order as indicated. If time and space are limited a five station circuit composed of sit-up, back extension, squat, overhead press, and biceps curl is recommended.

CHAPTER 5 References

Adamson, G. T. (1959). "Circuit Training." *Ergonomics* **2**:183–186.

Berger, R. A. (1962). "Effect of Varied Weight Training Programs on Strength." *Research Quarterly of the American Association for Health, Physical Education, and Recreation* **33**:168–181.

Berger, R. A., and Harris, M. W. (1966). "Effects of Various Repetitive Rates in Weight Training on Improvements in Strength and Endurance." *American Corrective Therapy Journal* **20**:205–207.

DeLorme, T., and Watkins, A. (1951). *Progressive Resistance Exercise.* Appleton, New York.

Jones, H. H. (1965). "The Valsalva Procedure: Its Clinical Importance to the Physical Therapist." *Journal of the American Physical Therapy Association* **45**:570–572.

Keegan, J. J. (1953). "Alterations of the Lumbar Curve Related to Posture and Seating." *Journal Bone Joint Surgery* **35A**:589–603.

Mathews, D. K., and Kruse, R. D. (1957). "Effects of Isometric and Isotonic Exercises on Elbow Flexor Muscle Group." *Research Quarterly of the American Association for Health, Physical Education, and Recreation* **28**:26–37.

Morgan, R. E., and Adamson, G. T. (1961). *Circuit Training.* Sportshelf & Soccer, New Rochelle, New York.

SIX/
Endurance

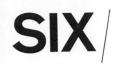

SIX/

One who has developed endurance has the ability to sustain intense activity for a period of time, to continue hard work, postpone fatigue, and recover rapidly. It has been common practice among exercise specialists to identify two types of endurance —local and general. Local endurance refers to the ability to sustain or repeat contraction in a single muscle or group of muscles. General endurance involves a sustaining of activity in many of the large muscles of the body and is usually referred to as cardiorespiratory or cardiovascular endurance. Actually, these two endurances are basically the same since they both depend upon adequate oxygen supply and strength in the working muscles.

Movements of the large antigravity muscles are especially important to functioning Man since it is on these muscles that the heaviest demand is placed in performance of most physical work, participation in sports, maintenance of an efficient erect posture, and protection of joints from injury. Movements of these large muscles also place the greatest stress on the cardiovascular system. It is exercise of these muscles which principally conditions the cardiovascular system thus aiding in the prevention of circulatory disease (Evang and Andersen, 1966).

I. AEROBIC AND ANAEROBIC PROCESSES

In Chapter Two, Huxley's sliding filament model of muscle contraction was discussed. This theory of contraction holds that actin and myosin filaments within a muscle fiber "slide" past each other and that this interaction between the two types of filaments causes a shortening of the entire fiber. The energy that causes the filaments to slide is provided by the breakdown of phosphagens [adenosine-triphosphate (ATP) and phosphocreatine (PC)], which is triggered by the release of acetylcholine at the neuromuscular junction. The total supply of phosphagens is small, but fortunately, it can be resynthesized and used over and over.

This resynthesis is brought about by supplying oxygen for the oxidation of foodstuffs (glucose and free fatty acids). The oxidation produces energy along with the associated waste products CO_2 and H_2O. The energy is used to resynthesize the split phosphagen. A limiting factor is the body's ability to keep a fresh supply of oxygen available. As long as enough O_2 is made available for the resynthesis of phosphagens, muscular work can go on indefinitely. The relative ability to supply oxygen *during* muscular contraction is called *aerobic capacity* (maximum oxygen consumption), and most exercise physiologists consider it to be the best indicator of a person's endurance.

If insufficient oxygen is made available through the aerobic processes, the body can utilize one other source of energy for resynthesis of the phosphagens. This source is the breakdown of glycogen to lactic acid (glycolysis). This process is called the *anaerobic mechanism*. However, lactic acid is a fatigue toxin, and once the maximum ability of the muscle to tolerate its accumulation has been reached, activity must be slowed to a level below which no additional glycolysis occurs. Otherwise, work must of necessity cease. After work stops, increased oxygen consumption is maintained in order to resynthesize lactic acid to glycogen. This repays the so-called O_2 debt. The aerobic and anaerobic utilization of oxygen is pictured schematically in Figure 6.1.

The renowned Italian physiologist, Margaria (1968) has summarized biochemical events occurring in muscle as follows:

$$\text{PG} \underset{b}{\overset{a}{\rightleftharpoons}} \text{ADP} + 2\text{P} + \text{C} + \text{EN}_P \nearrow \overset{W}{\underset{}{}}$$

$$\text{Food} + O_2 \overset{c}{\rightarrow} CO_2 + H_2O + \text{En}_o$$

$$\text{Glycogen} \underset{e}{\overset{d}{\rightleftharpoons}} \text{Lactic Acid} + \text{En}_L$$

where PG is phosphagen (ATP and CP), W is work produced, En is energy (P from phosphagen splitting, O from oxidation, and L from glycolysis). In reaction

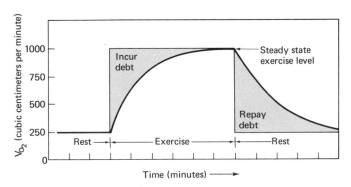

FIGURE 6.1   The Time Course of Oxygen Consumption during Exercise and Recovery. If the exercise is strenuous the O_2 consumed during the exercise (V_{O_2}) ordinarily lags behind the demand. Therefore, part of the energy needed must be provided through anaerobic means, and an O_2 debt is contracted. After exercise ceases, the O_2 consumption remains elevated for a time in order to repay the debt and resynthesize the phosphagens that have been broken down. The volume of debt incurred and repaid can be evaluated by measuring the area of the shaded regions (From Brown, A. C. and Brengelmann, G. (1965). "Energy Metabolism," *In Physiology and Biophysics* (19 ed.), (T. C. Ruch, and H. D. Patton, eds.), pp. 1030–1049. Saunders, Philadelphia, Pennsylvania).

a, phosphagens (ATP + PC) split to form adenosine-diphosphate (ADP) and creatine (C) plus two free phosphate molecules. This provides energy (En_p) for activation of the actin and myosin filaments (work). Either reaction c or d provides the energy for resynthesis (reaction b). If it has been necessary to call upon anaerobic energy sources, resynthesis of glycogen (reaction e) is provided by continuation of increased oxidation after exercise (reaction c).*

Although there is evidence to indicate that physical training increases the available stores of muscle protein, ATP (Gordon, 1967), and glycogen stores (Astrand, 1956) and increases one's tolerance to lactic acid accumulation (Knehr et al., 1942), oxygen supply is by far the key factor in endurance (Chapman and Mitchell, 1965).

II. RESPIRATION AND THE SUPPLY OF OXYGEN

Respiration and circulation, modified by nervous and chemical mechanisms, are the primary functions involved in insuring an adequate supply of oxygen to the working muscles. Atmospheric air contains approximately 21 percent O_2, and this is the source from which, ultimately, muscles and other body cells are supplied. Approximately 79 percent of the remaining atmospheric air is nitrogen (N_2). Carbon dioxide (CO_2) and other gases account for less than 1 percent of the total mixture. The total pressure exerted by this gaseous mixture is 760 millimeters of mercury (Hg) at sea level. Since O_2 makes up 21 percent of the total pressure or 160 millimeters of Hg, this fraction of the total pressure is called the *partial pressure of oxygen* (P_{O_2}).

The lungs are responsible for supplying the body with fresh O_2 and also for removing excess CO_2 and

---

* It should be noted that the above reactions have been presented in a highly simplified manner. Several intermediate stages are involved. The reader who is interested in a detailed discussion of these should consult the sections on metabolism in a good textbook of physiology such as Guyton (1966) or Ruch and Patton (1965) or see Gollnick and King (1969).

H_2O. Air is brought into the lungs by action of the diaphragm and the mechanical deformation of the rib cage by the external intercostal muscles. Contraction of these muscles increases the size of the chest cavity. This decreases the pressure of the gas in the lungs according to Boyle's Law causing it to drop below that of the atmospheric pressure outside the body. Air then rushes into the lungs due to the difference in pressure (pressure gradient) (See Figure 6.2).

By the time the oxygen reaches the air sacs (alveoli) of the lungs, its partial pressure has been reduced to approximately 100 millimeters of Hg due to mixing with air having lower O_2 concentrations. The lung–capillary membrane is only three cells in thickness, and O_2 diffuses easily into the blood-stream, again due to a pressure gradient (See Figures 6.3 and 6.4). O_2 partial pressure in the venous blood returning to the lungs from the body is approximately 40 millimeters of Hg. This blood picks up enough new oxygen in the lungs so that it has a P_{O_2} equal to approximately 100 millimeters of Hg when it leaves them. From the lungs the blood returns to the left side of the heart from which it is pumped to all parts of the body. A schematic representation of circulation is presented in Figure 6.5. Most of the oxygen entering the bloodstream from the lungs combines with hemoglobin, a protein found in the red blood cell. The circulation of the red blood cell serves as the major O_2 transporting mechanism.

Due to the oxidative processes discussed earlier in the chapter, P_{O_2} in the muscle cells is low. This creates a pressure gradient between the blood in the capillaries and the muscle tissues, causing hemoglobin to release oxygen, which diffuses into the muscle cells.

Carbon dioxide produced through the oxidation processes must be removed from the body. This, too, is accomplished by simple diffusion. P_{CO_2} (partial pressure of CO_2) builds up to approximately 48 millimeters of Hg in the muscle tissue due to oxidation. P_{CO_2} in the blood coming from the heart is about 40 millimeters of Hg. This pressure gradient results in diffusion of CO_2 into the blood as it passes through

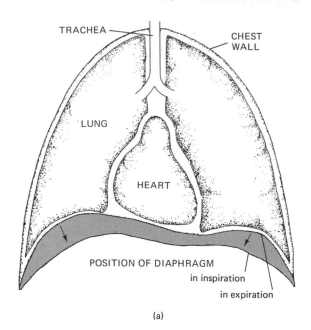

POSITION OF DIAPHRAGM

in inspiration

in expiration

(a)

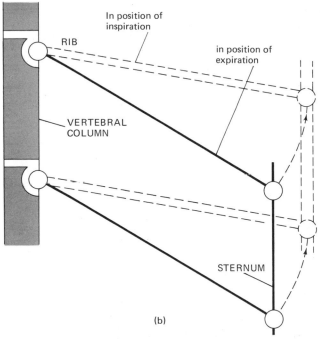

(b)

FIGURE 6.2   Lung Space Changes during Respiration. (a) shows the contraction of the diaphragm during inspiration causes it to descend. The resultant increase in chest volume is indicated in black. (b) shows the elevation of the front ends of the ribs, or of the sternum to which the ribs are attached. This causes an increase in the front–back diameter of the chest. Both the above movements allow air to rush into the lungs. The reverse occurs during expiration (From Carlson, A. J. and Johnson, V. (1948). *The Machinery of the Body*, p. 231. University of Chicago Press, Chicago, Illinois. © Copyright 1948 by The University of Chicago Press).

the capillaries. It is then transported through the right side of the heart to the lungs. Because P_{CO_2} in in the lung alveoli is only 40 millimeters of Hg, the excess diffuses from the blood into the alveoli where it is removed from the body by expiration.

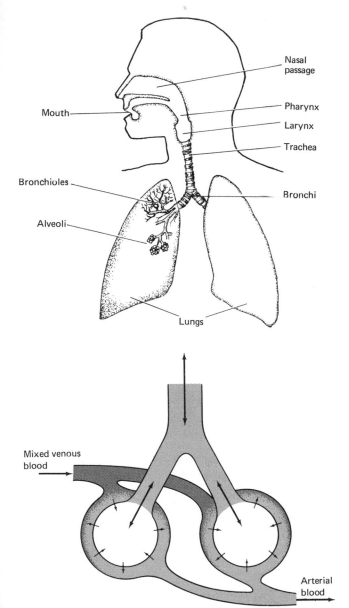

Nasal passage

Pharynx

Mouth

Larynx

Trachea

Bronchioles

Bronchi

Alveoli

Lungs

Mixed venous blood

Arterial blood

FIGURE 6.3   Schematic Representation of the Respiratory Apparatus. Oxygen enters the mouth and nose, passes through the trachea to the lungs, where it diffuses from the alveoli into the bloodstream. Carbon dioxide diffusion follows a reverse path (From Mathews, D. K., Stacy, R. W., and Hoover, G. N. (1964). *Physiology of Muscular Activity and Exercise.* Ronald Press, New York. Copyright © 1964.).

FIGURE 6.4   Schematic of the Lungs and Pulmonary Circulation. The rounded areas represent alveoli; the shaded tubes leading to them represent all of the conducting airways. Mixed venous blood (dark) flows through vessels in intimate contact with ventilated alveoli and becomes arterial blood (light). The fine arrows represent the transfer of O_2 and CO_2 between gas and blood (From Comroe, J. H. (1965). *Physiology of Respiration*, p. 11. Year Book Medical Publishers, Chicago, Illinois).

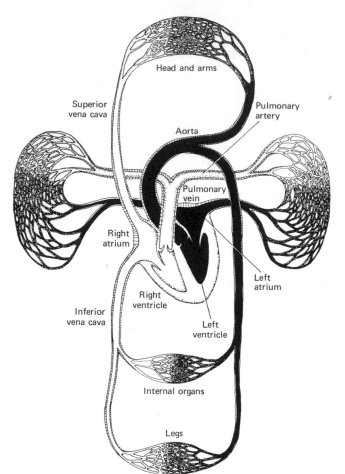

FIGURE 6.5   Schematic of Heart and Blood Circulation. Lighter shaded areas represent mixed venous blood. Darker areas show parts containing arterial (oxygenated) blood. (From Wiggers, C. J. "The Heart." *Scientific American* **196**(5):74–87. Copyright © May, 1957 by Scientific American. All rights reserved.)

Expiration is accomplished by relaxation of the diaphragm and external intercostals plus contraction of the internal intercostals, abdominal muscles, and some shoulder muscles (See Figure 6.2). These actions decrease the size of the chest cavity, thereby compressing the enclosed gas and raising its pressure above that of atmospheric air (Boyle's Law). This causes a pressure gradient toward the outside of the body, and air rushes out of the lungs. Figure 6.6 is a schematic presentation of the entire process of O_2 supply and CO_2 removal.

III. MAXIMUM OXYGEN CONSUMPTION LEVEL AND ITS IMPORTANCE TO ENDURANCE

During normal resting activities the processes illustrated in Figure 6.6 supply approximately 225 milliliters* of O_2 per minute, and they remove the accumulated CO_2. In order to exercise intensely, O_2 deliverly and CO_2 removal must be speeded greatly. These increased demands are met primarily by greater release of O_2 from hemoglobin at the tissue level and a speed up of circulation and respiration.

At rest, hemoglobin releases at the tissues approximately 25 percent of the oxygen bound to it. During strenuous exercise as much as 75–80 percent of the O_2 is released. This response is dependent upon the partial pressure of oxygen in the muscle tissues and is illustrated graphically by the classical oxyhemoglobin dissociation curve of Figure 6.7. This increased release from hemoglobin can triple the oxygen supply to the muscles. The cardiac output at rest (volume of blood pumped by the heart in one minute) is approximately 5000 milliliters. Strenuous exercise can cause this output to reach 25000 milliliters, five times the resting level. The cardiac output is increased by raising the heart rate from approximately 70 per minute to 180 per minute and by increasing the stroke volume (amount of blood pumped per heartbeat) from approximately 70 to 140 milliliters (Guyton, 1966).

These combined mechanisms—greater release of O_2 by hemoglobin and increased cardiac output—can provide a 15-fold increase in O_2 delivery to the tissues. The O_2 supply may thus increase from 225 to 3375 milliliters per minute. This 3375 milliliters of O_2 per minute approximates the average maximum oxygen consumption for a young adult male (Shephard, 1966; Cumming, 1967).

As previously noted, maximum oxygen consumption is considered by most exercise physiologists to be the best indicator of physical fitness (endurance). It is defined as the maximum amount of O_2 that one

* A milliliter is 1/1000 of a liter, which is slightly larger than a quart in volume. Therefore 225 milliliters is approximately 1/4 quart by volume.

Physiological process	Ventilation	Diffusion
Organ system	Lungs	
Physiological quantities	TLV, VC, MBC	
Functional capacities	$\dot{V}_E$	D_L
Overall O_2 Transport	$\dot{V}_{O_2}$	

FIGURE 6.6 Schematic Illustration of the Oxygen Transport System with Measures of Quantities and Functional Capacities of the Important Components. Arrows pointing right indicate direction of O_2 diffusion, and arrows pointing left the direction of CO_2 diffusion. TLV is total lung volume; VC is vital capacity; MBC is maximum breathing capacity; THb is total circulating hemoglobin; Hb is hemoglobin concentration; HV is heart volume; F_{max} is maximum heart rate; $\dot{V}_E$ is minute volume of ventilation; D_L is lung diffusing capacity; $\dot{Q}$ is cardiac output; SV is

can take *into* the body and *utilize* for oxidation per minute. As we have already seen, this is the primary determinant of ability to sustain work. It is best measured by having the person walk to exhaustion on a motor driven treadmill as samples of expired air are analyzed for their volume and O_2 content (Figure 1.2). The obtained result is expressed in milliliters per minute per kilogram* body weight. This is a time-consuming and expensive process.

---

* A kilogram is 2.2 pounds.

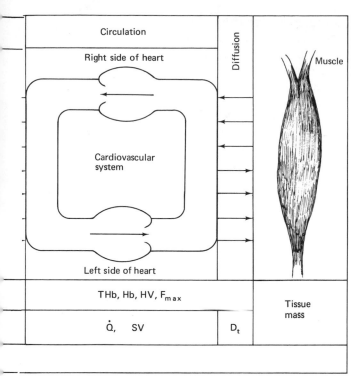

stroke volume of the heart; D_t is tissue diffusing capacity, $\dot{V}_{O_2}$ is maximum oxygen intake (Adapted from Holmgren, A. (1967).

"Cardiorespiratory determinants of cardiovascular fitness."

Canadian Medical Association Journal **96**:697–702).

Therefore, it is not applicable outside the research laboratory. Fortunately, some good practical approximations to the procedure have been recently established, and these can be used by the individual wishing to estimate his maximum oxygen intake (see Chapter Seven).

In Figure 6.8 endurance (maximum oxygen consumption) is viewed as a continuum extending from very low (about 20 milliliters per minute per kilogram) to very high (about 80 milliliters per minute per kilogram). A person's maximum displacement toward the right of the continuum is determined by heredity, for example, the better his genetic stock the farther to the right he will be able to go. Note that this is his maximum attainable displacement. His environment and/or his behavior will determine how closely he approaches this maximum. Environmental and behavioral factors will be limiting since the inherited potential assumes a perfectly favorable environment and behavior.

Environmental factors which limit achievement of the maximum potential include, for example, disabling accidents, debilitating diseases, and residence in unfavorable environments. Affecting behavior factors include smoking, which limits lung diffusion, accumulation of excess body fat through

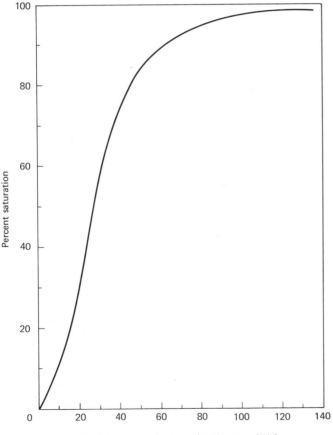

FIGURE 6.7   The O_2–Hemoglobin Dissociation Curve. When the partial pressure (P_{O_2}) of oxygen is high, it combines readily with hemoglobin in the blood. This is the normal situation in the lungs (right-hand portion of curve). When O_2 partial pressure is low, such as in the muscle tissue, it is readily released from the hemoglobin (left-hand part of curve). Drops in P_{O_2} below 40 millimeters of Hg in the muscles cause rapid release of O_2 from the hemoglobin. During rest P_{O_2} in the muscle cells is about 35 millimeters of Hg. During strenuous exercise it drops much lower, resulting in a greatly increased O_2 supply to the muscle. Total O_2 supply can be increased threefold simply by operation of the mechanism. (Graph from Mathews, D. K., Stacy, R. W. and Hoover, G. N. (1964). *Physiology of Muscular Activity and Exercise.* Ronald Press, New York. Copyright © 1964.)

poor dietary and exercise habits, and decrease in other functions due to sedentary living. Behavior is the more important of the two factors since, barring unforeseen circumstances, one can control his environment to a great degree.

Figure 6.9 shows the effect of age and activity upon the maximum oxygen consumption. The respiratory and circulatory functions reach a peak at about 16 to 20 years of age. Thereafter they gradually decline due to a progressive development of

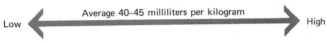

Low ⟵——— Average 40–45 milliliters per kilogram ———⟶ High

20 milliliters per kilogram
Lung disease
Sedentary habits
Circulatory disease
Poor nutrition

80 milliliters per kilogram
Participation in endurance sports
Good genetic stock
Excellent nutrition

FIGURE 6.8   Maximum O₂ Consumption (Endurance) Continuum. Lowest values are around 20 milliliters per kilogram per minute and are a result of lung disease, sedentary habits, circulatory disease, poor nutrition, etc. Average for adult males is 40–45 milliliters per kilogram per minute. Highest known values (80 milliliters per kilogram per minute) have been recorded in endurance athletes (skiers, long distance runners).

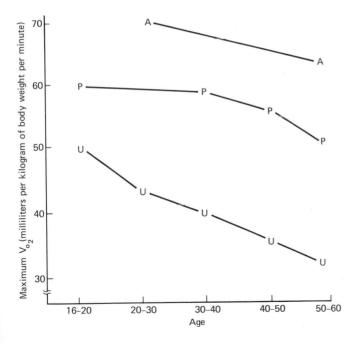

FIGURE 6.9   Relationship of Physical Work Capacity (Maximum Oxygen Consumption) to Age and Activity Level. A, male athletes; P, active male nonathletes; U, sedentary (untrained) males (Based on data of Shephard (1966) and Cumming (1967)).

inelasticity in the lungs and arterial tree, overweight, and weakened general musculature. Much of this deterioration can be delayed or reversed by regular physical activity and good health habits (for example, proper nutrition, avoidance of smoking, proper sleep). The effects of regular physical activity are readily apparent in Figure 6.9. It is possible for a man in the sixth or seventh decade of life to have an endurance level equivalent to that of the *average* man of 20 to 30 years old.

Scientific evidence suggests that regular physical activity favorably affects several of the functional capacities involved in supplying oxygen to the muscles (Astrand, 1956; Brouha, 1962; Consolazio *et al.*, 1963; Andersen, 1968). Observation of Figure 6.6 shows that maximum oxygen consumption depends on several physiological quantities and capacities. The most important quantities are total lung capacity (TLC), total hemoglobin (THb), hemoglobin concentration (Hb), blood volume (BV), heart volume (HV), and maximum attainable heart rate (F_{max}). Changes in these quantities actually determine changes in the functional capacities of maximal pulmonary ventilation ($\dot{V}_E$) lung diffusing capacity (D_L) maximal cardiac output ($\dot{Q}$), and diffusing capacity for oxygen at the tissue level (D_t). Stroke volume (SV) changes are probably due to neurological changes, and favorable changes in tissue mass are brought about by reduced caloric intake and/or burning of stored fat for fuel in reaction c of phosphagen breakdown on page 109. (See Chapter Eight for a discussion of oxidation of fat in the body).

IV. CHRONIC EFFECTS OF EXERCISE

A. Heart Size, Weight, and Vascularization

Research evidence from both human and animal studies suggests that the heart muscle itself is favorably affected by exercise. In an attempt to assess the effect of habitual physical activity on the heart, Poupa and Rakusan (1966) compared wild animals with domesticated ones of the same species. They summarized their results as follows:

(1) In wild or athletic animals the heart is larger relative to the body than in nonathletic or domesticated ones.
(2) The capillary density in the hearts of athletic or wild animals is larger than in nonathletic or domesticated ones.
(3) The number of muscle cells per unit heart mass in athletic or wild animals is larger than in nonathletic or domesticated ones.
(4) The cardiac cells in athletic or wild animals are smaller than in nonathletic or domesticated ones.

Results similar to the above have been obtained by other investigators (Andersen, 1968). Limited research on man has yielded findings consistent with those on animals. Figure 6.10 and Table 6.1 both indicate that active men have larger heart volumes than inactive men. Table 6.1 also indicates that the heart volume is related to the degree of activity, for example, the more active individuals have relatively larger heart volumes.

Table 6.1
Heart Volume Estimated from Areas of Heart Shadow*

| Subjects | N | Heart volume (milliliters) | |
		$\overline{X}$	Range
Normals	67	790	490–1080
Wrestlers and high jumpers	30	782	610– 920
Swimmers, soccer players, and tennis players	86	876	605–1130
Skiers, long distance runners, and swimmers	66	923	645–1180
Professional cyclists	18	1104	880–1460

* Reprinted from Andersen, 1968; original data after Reindell et al., 1960.

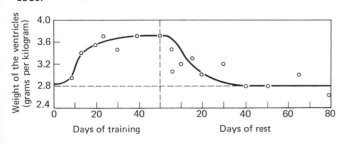

FIGURE 6.10   The Size of the Heart as Affected by Training (Andersen, 1968, original data from Reindell et al., 1960).

B. Circulatory Functions

Other favorable effects that exercise has on the circulatory capacity can be seen by comparing the differences between sedentary and active individuals as in Table 6.2. Each of the illustrated circulatory measures (except for maximum heart rate) is seen to be higher in the active men. The lower maximum heart rate of the active person has been interpreted as indicating a functional reserve that it is not necessary to call upon (Andersen, 1968).

Table 6.2
Circulatory Differences between Sedentary and Active Males*

Circulatory measure	Sedentary	Active
Cardiac output (rest–upright) (liters per minute)	5.85	6.61
Stroke volume (rest) (millilters per minute)	70	103
Heart rate (rest) (beats per minute)	84	64
Blood volume (liters)	5.7	7.5
Total Hb (grams per kilogram body weight)	10.3	14.0
Cardiac output (maximum exercise) (liters per minute)	22.8	27.9
Heart rate (maximum) (beats per minute)	198	180
Stroke volume (maximum) (milliliters per minute)	116	162

* Data adapted from Carlsten and Grimby (1966) and Andersen (1968).

C. Ventilatory Functions

Differences in ventilatory functions among individuals in relation to physical training have been less well-investigated and described than circulatory functions. However, many workers have reported that physically active persons exhibit favorable differences.

A considerable volume of research literature is available demonstrating that well-trained persons generally exhibit higher vital capacities than untrained persons (Bainbridge, 1931; Welham and Behnke, 1942; Stuart and Collings, 1959). P. O. Astrand, a world famous Swedish exercise physiologist, has stated, "The vital capacity must be regarded as one of the many factors determining the working capacity. A certain connection with the maximal oxygen intake is justifiable, as there is a great dependence between vital capacity and the maximal tidal air during exercise" (Astrand, 1952).

It is obvious that any improvement of the individual's ability to move oxygen through the lungs and into the bloodstream would improve the overall working capacity. Several factors are involved in this mechanism. The maximum minute volume is increased by increases in the depth and frequency of breathing. The efficiency of the ventilation is also increased as evidenced by a higher ventilation equivalent in the trained person (Schneider and Crampton, 1940). This apparent increased extraction of oxygen from the inspired air implies a greater lung diffusing capacity.

D. Body Composition

Another factor contributing to higher working capacity is increased muscle mass especially in relation to the total body weight. Percentage lean body weight* has been shown to be an important component in physical fitness (Falls *et al.*, 1965). In addition, lower fat-free body mass* has been offered as a possible explanation for the fact that women have a lower working capacity than men (Astrand, 1956).

CHAPTER 6   References

Andersen, K. L. (1968). "The Cardiovascular System in Exercise." *In Exercise Physiology* (H. B. Falls, ed.), pp. 79–128. Academic Press, New York.

Astrand, P. O. (1952). "Experimental Studies of Physical Working Capacity. *In Relation to Sex and Age.* Munksgaard, Copenhagen.

Astrand, P. O. (1952). *Experimental Studies in Physical Working Capacity in Relation to Sex and Age.* Munksgaard, Copenhagen.

---

* See Chapter Eight, page 156 for a discussion of body composition relationships to fitness.

Bainbridge, F. A. (1931). *The Physiology of Muscular Exercise.* Longmans, Green, New York.

Brouha, L. (1962). "Physiology of Training, including Age and Sex Differences." *Journal of Sports Medicine and Physical Fitness* **2**:3–11.

Carlsten, A., and Grimby, G. (1966). *The Circulatory Response to Muscular Exercise in Man.* Thomas, Springfield, Illinois.

Chapman, C. B., and Mitchell, J. H. (1965). "The Physiology of Exercise." *Scientific American* **212**(5): 88–96.

Consolazio, C. F., Johnson, R. E., and Pecora, L. J. (1963). *Physiological Measurements of Metabolic Functions in Man.* McGraw-Hill, New York.

Cumming, G. R. (1967). "Current Levels of Fitness." *Canadian Medical Association Journal* **96**:868–877.

Evang, K., and Andersen, K. L. (1966). *Physical Activity in Health and Disease.* Williams and Wilkins, Baltimore, Maryland.

Falls, H. B., Ismail, A. H., MacLeod, D. F., Wiebers, J. E., Christian, J. E., and Kessler, M. V. (1965). "Development of Physical Fitness Test Batteries by Factor Analysis Techniques." *Journal of Sports Medicine and Physical Fitness* **4**:185–197.

Gollnick, P. D., and King, D. W. (1969). "Energy Release in the Muscle Cell." *Medicine and Science in Sports* **1**:23–31.

Gordon, E. E. (1967). "Anatomical and Biochemical Adaptations of Muscle to Different Exercises." *Journal American Medical Association* **201**:755–758.

Guyton, A. C. (1966). *Textbook of Medical Physiology.* Saunders, Philadelphia, Pennsylvania.

Knehr, C. A., Dill, D. B., and Neufeld, W. (1942). "Training and Its Effects on Man at Rest and at Work." *American Journal of Physiology* **136**:148–156.

Margaria, R. (1968). "Energy Sources for Aerobic and Anaerobic Work." In *Physiological Aspects of Sports and Physical Fitness* (B. Balke, ed.), pp. 20–25. Athletic Institute, Chicago, Illinois.

Poupa, O., and Rakusan, K. (1966). "The Terminal Microcirculatory Bed in the Heart of Athletic and Nonathletic Animals." *In Physical Activity in Health and Disease* (K. Evang and K. L. Andersen, eds.), pp. 18–29. Williams and Wilkins, Baltimore, Maryland.

Reindell, H., Klepzig, H., Steim, H., Musshoff, K., Roskamm, H., and Schildge, E. (1960). *Herz Kreislaufkrankeiten und Sport.* Barth, Munich, Germany.

Ruch, T. C., and Patton, H. D. (1965). *Physiology and Biophysics.* Saunders, Philadelphia, Pennsylvania.

Schneider, E. C., and Crampton, C. B. (1940). "A Comparison of Some Respiratory and Circulatory Reactions of Athletes and Nonathletes." *American Journal of Physiology* **129**:165–170.

Shephard, R. J. (1966). "World Standards of Cardiorespiratory Performance." *Archives of Environmental Health* **13**:664–672.

Stuart, D. G., and Collings, W. D. (1959). "Comparison of Vital Capacity and Maximum Breathing Capacity of Athletes and Nonathletes." *Journal of Applied Physiology* **14**:507–509.

Welham, W. C., and Behnke, A. R. (1942). "The Specific Gravity of Healthy Men. Body Weight— Volume and Other Physical Characteristics of Exceptional Athletes and of Naval Personnel." *Journal of the American Medical Association* **118**:498–501.

SEVEN/
Endurance
Training
Procedures

SEVEN /

Many of the benefits to be derived from regular physical activity have been described. These include improved efficiency for the circulatory, respiratory, neuromuscular, and other systems. As a result of training one is less likely to suffer from chronic debilitating problems such as cardiovascular disease and obesity.

In order to obtain maximum benefit from exercise, one must regularly engage in a systematic planned program of physical activity contributing to endurance. This chapter presents some suggestions for such a regular program.

I. PREREQUISITES

Before beginning any program of physical activity one should obtain a thorough medical examination to be sure that there are no contraindications for a strenuous exercise. Exercise may be one of the most severe stresses that can be placed on the human organism. Although the healthy person cannot be harmed by physical activity, an already existing heart disease, a joint injury, or similar condition might be aggravated. If such a condition does exist the physician can then recommend the type of activities which are appropriate and those to be avoided.

Rest is important as a restorative mechanism. During sleep the body should have sufficient time to recover from the day's ravages. It is impossible to prescribe the proper amount of sleep that an individual needs since these needs vary quite widely. Some can get by on four to five hours of sleep, while others may need eight to ten. Through experience one should be able to determine his sleep needs. Often less sleep is needed than might be expected. If nutrition is adequate, emotional tension is light, and there is no reason to suspect organic disease, but one feels tired after arising in the morning, it is likely that sleep has been inadequate. If this is the case, sleep should be increased.

II. SELF-TESTING

Before beginning the endurance training program an assessment should be made of one's condition in comparison to established standards for fitness. This will satisfy a natural curiosity and also enable the participant to better plan the type of program he needs.

In Chapter Six it was established that maximum oxygen consumption is the best measure of one's endurance fitness. It was also pointed out that this measurement involved time-consuming laboratory procedures unavailable to the average individual in determining his fitness level. Fortunately, accurate short cut procedures are available. One of these is outlined by Cooper (1968a). Based on his own work and on the work of a few other exercise physiologists, Dr. Kenneth H. Cooper has devised a 12-minute field test (Aerobics Test) that will allow a good approximation of one's maximum oxygen consumption. Dr. Cooper has further established standards that indicate whether one's fitness is excellent, good, fair, poor, or very poor in relation to the adult male population (See Table 7.1). The test is simple. All one need do is determine how far he can go by running

Table 7.1
Standards for Cooper's 12-Minute Field Test of Fitness

Fitness category	Distance covered (miles)	Equivalent O$_2$ consumption (milliliters per minute)
I Very poor	less than 1.0	28.0 or less
II Poor	1.0–1.24	28.1–34
III Fair	1.25–1.49	34.1–42
IV Good	1.50–1.74*	42.1–52
V Excellent	1.75 or more	52.1 or more

* For men 35 years of age, 1.40 miles in 12 minutes is consistent with the good fitness category. (Adapted from K. H. Cooper, "A Means of Assessing Maximal Oxygen Intake." *Journal of the American Medical Association* **203**:201–204 (1968). © American Medical Association). One should note that the Fair category here represents no better than the average for the untrained male of 20 to 30 years of age from Figure 6.9 of Chapter Six.

and walking in a 12-minute time period.

This test has a sound scientific base. It is an outgrowth of research work done by Cooper (1968b) and by Balke (1963). Both investigators correlated the results of running with maximum oxygen intakes determined from treadmill work. Balke found that estimates from running were usually within ±10 percent of actual values, and Cooper obtained a correlation coefficient of 0.897, which is very high (Figure 7.1). Balke experimented with several different running distances and concluded that a running test that lasted at least 12 minutes but less than 20 was optimum. Cooper extended the work of Balke in developing the 12-minute test. Running for at least 12 minutes insures that most of the work is done aerobically rather than anaerobically. Figure 7.2 shows graphically the aerobic–anaerobic relationship for runs of various distances. It is readily apparent that as the length of running increases, a larger and larger percentage of the work is done aerobically, giving a truer picture of the functioning of the oxygen transport mechanisms.

III. SELECTING THE EXERCISE PROGRAM: INTENSITY AND CALORIC EXPENDITURE

Once one has determined where he stands on the fitness scale, he will need to determine what type of fitness program is best for him. If he scores in Categories IV or V on the Aerobics Test, he may merely wish to maintain his present condition. However, he may wish to improve it, and there is no reason why he cannot. Examination of Figure 6.9 readily indicates that individuals who regularly participate in sport activities score well above Category V in oxygen consumption. If the score is in Categories I, II, or III, there is considerable room for improvement up to a more desirable fitness level.

The basic consideration in selecting exercise to include in the program is that it be strenuous enough to produce a training effect. Cooper (1968a) has laid down two basic principles in this regard,

(1) "If the exercise is vigorous enough to produce a sustained heart rate of 150 beats per minute or more, the training effect benefits begin about five minutes after the exercise starts and continue as long as the exercise is performed.

(2) If the exercise is not vigorous enough to produce or sustain a heart rate of 150 beats per minute, but is still demanding oxygen, the exercise must be continued considerably longer than five minutes, the total period of time depending on the oxygen consumed."

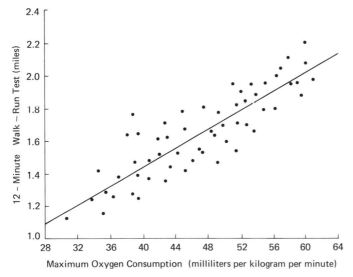

FIGURE 7.1 Correlation between Maximal Oxygen Consumption and a 12-Minute Run–Walk Performance in Normal Males. 115 normal males age 17–52 (Redrawn from Cooper, K. H. (1968). "A Means of Assessing Maximal Oxygen Intake." *Journal of the American Medical Association* **203:**201–204.)

These statements are partially confirmed by the work of Jackson (1967), Karvonen et al., (1957), and Karvonen (1959).

The level to which one's heart rate rises during any given exercise is dependent upon his relative physical fitness. The poorer conditioned he is, the less strenuous will be the exercise needed to raise his pulse rate to 150. It might require a mile run in less than 5 minutes to raise the pulse rate of an athlete such as Jim Ryun to 150, whereas, the man who is sedentary in his habits might need only to walk at a brisk pace to reach the same pulse rate.

This brings out another basic principle. It is possible for the sedentary, poorly conditioned man to start out with relatively light exercise and still receive a training benefit. He might take several weeks to work up to more strenuous activities.

It is quite easy for one to determine what level his pulse rate assumes during a particular activity. All he need do is palpate with a finger the radial artery located on the inner, thumb side of his wrist. He can then feel the pulsations as the heart pumps blood into the arterial tree. Since it is very difficult to do this while one is exercising, it must be done after the exercise stops. The pulse rate drops very rapidly after cessation of exercise, so the count should be taken *immediately* after the exercise for only the first 10 seconds. This count can be multiplied by 6 to obtain the rate per minute.

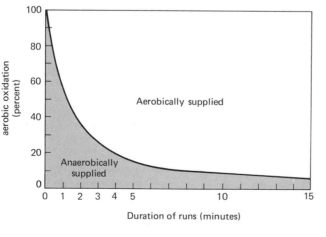

FIGURE 7.2   The Relative Role of Anaerobic and Aerobic Oxidation for Supplying the Total Amounts of Oxygen Required during Best Effort Runs of Defined Time Intervals. Shaded area represents the proportion of total energy requirements that must be supplied anaerobically for runs of various duration (From Balke, 1963).

All physical activities require that the body increase its oxygen consumption in order to supply the muscles performing the work. The amount of oxygen required for a particular type of activity is directly proportional to the number of contractions occurring within the muscles. Each time six oxygen molecules are oxidized with one glucose molecule, energy is produced. The basic unit in which energy is expressed is the kilocalorie (Calorie). Each liter of oxygen that is oxidized produces slightly less than 5 kilocalories of energy. This is called the *caloric equivalent* of oxygen. It is this caloric equivalent that is used to express the intensity of an activity and not the actual oxygen consumption. For instance, an average size man sitting at ease requires 1.6 kilocalories per minute, while one cycling at 13 miles per hour requires 11.1 kilocalories per minute (Passmore and Durnin, 1955). Tables comparing various sport activities in this manner are readily available (Figure 7.3).

It is obvious that activities involving greater caloric expenditures, if they can be sustained for more than five minutes, will produce the greatest training bene-

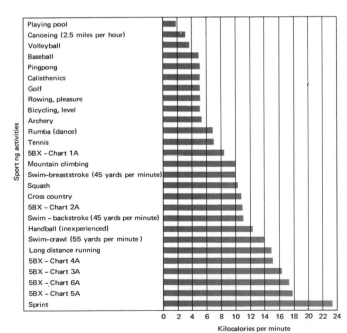

FIGURE 7.3 The Kilocalorie Energy Expenditure per Minute for Typical Sporting Activities (From Banister and Brown, 1968).

fits since they require a higher level of functioning from the oxygen transport system. Exercises such as sprinting (Figure 7.3) which require kilocalorie expenditures in excess of 20 per minute are over too soon to produce the significant training effect that has been discussed. One cannot maintain the high rate of energy expenditure long enough. This is why sprint swimmers, soccer players, and tennis players have smaller hearts than skiers, long distance swimmers, long distance runners and professional cyclists (Table 6.1). Although their activities require short bursts of high energy expenditure, it does not remain high long enough to produce a large endurance training effect on heart size.

Cooper (1968a) has rated physical activities somewhat differently than in Figure 7.3. He has established a point system in connection with his 12-minute test. He claims that one must accumulate 30 points per week in order to receive a training effect equivalent to Category IV or V. The energy expenditure involved is equivalent to running a mile in less than eight minutes six days a week. Table 7.2 presents equivalent rates for other types of activity.

The individual who initially scores lower than Category IV or V on the 12-minute test may find his level of condition too low for him to pleasurably participate at the intensities of exercise outlined in Table 7.2. If this is the case, he will want to exercise initially at a lower intensity and gradually work up to the level of Table 7.2. One whose fitness is already at or above Categories IV and V may want to choose a higher intensity than those in Table 7.2 in order to improve his endurance level.

Another way of classifying physical activities is in terms of the oxygen requirement in milliliters per kilogram of body weight per minute (Falls, 1969). Table 7.3 lists some common activities and their oxygen requirements.

The individual may obtain a good estimate of his own maximum oxygen intake from Table 7.1. This should be used as a guide in choosing activities for the development of endurance. If he is going to participate for only a few minutes he should choose an

Table 7.2
Rates of Activity Sufficient to Produce
a Significant Aerobic Training Effect †

Running	
1.0 mile	6.5–8 minutes
1.5 miles	15–18 minutes
2.0 miles	20–24 minutes
Swimming	
400 yards	Under 6:40 minutes
500 yards	Under 8:20 minutes
600 yards	10–15 minutes
Cycling	
4.0 miles	Under 12 minutes
5.0 miles	15–20 minutes
Walking	
2.5 miles	36:14–30:00 minutes
3.0 miles	43:23–36:00 minutes
Stationary Running*	
60–70 steps per minute	20 minutes
70–80 steps per minute	17.5 minutes
80–90 steps per minute	12.5 minutes
Handball/squash/basketball	35 minutes
Golf	27 holes
Skating	75 minutes
Tennis (singles)	3 sets
Volleyball	75 minutes

* Count only when the left foot hits the floor. Feet must be lifted at least eight inches from the floor. (Adapted from *Aerobics* by Kenneth H. Cooper, M.D., copyright © 1969 by Kenneth H. Cooper and Kevin Brown and published by M. Evans and Co., Inc. of New York.)

† In order to obtain the desired training effect the activity durations listed above should be repeated five to six times per week.

activity with an oxygen requirement very close to his own maximum. This will insure a heart rate of at least 150 per minute during the exercise. If, on the other hand, he anticipates that he will participate for one hour or longer, he should choose an activity with an O_2 requirement that is about one-half or slightly more of his maximum oxygen consumption. Research has shown that sustained participation (one hour or more) in activities requiring more than about 50 percent of one's maximum O_2 consumption is likely to result in physiological strain (sore muscles, strained

Table 7.3
Oxygen Requirements of Some Common Sport Activities*

Activity	O_2 requirement†	Energy expenditure (kilocalories per minute)
Volleyball	less than 10.5	less than 4.0
Baseball Tennis Dance Calisthenics Golf	10.5 to 21.0	4.0–7.5
Squash Handball	21.0–28.5	7.5–10.0
Jogging Swim—back stroke Swim—breast stroke	28.5–35.5	10–12.5
Running Swim—crawl	above 35.5	12.5–15.0

* Adapted from Falls, 1969.
† Values are given in milliliters O_2 per kilogram of body weight per minute.

tendons, undue fatigue, etc.) (Banister and Brown, 1968; Falls, 1969).

As an example, let's take the case of an individual who does 1.40 miles on the Aerobics Test. He would estimate from Table 7.1 that his maximum O_2 consumption is 38 milliliters per kilogram per minute. For short term activity he might choose running or brisk swimming as a conditioning activity (Table 7.3). For longer duration participation, he would want to choose an activity with an O_2 requirement of about 19 to 20 milliliters per minute. Tennis, dance, or calisthenics would be in this category.

IV. RELATIVE MERITS OF VARIOUS PHYSICAL ACTIVITIES

This chapter has emphasized that in order for a physical activity to contribute a significant training effect, it must cause the pulse rate to reach a level of 150 for five or more minutes. The training benefit accrues for the length of time that the exercise is extended beyond five minutes. Jogging, swimming, and cycling are excellent in this respect.

Activities such as handball, tennis, basketball, and circuit training (Chapter Five) are not as good, although they may require high energy expenditures for brief periods. A good deal of *resting* occurs during these sports due to lulls in the activity. This causes the *average* sustained heart rate to be somewhat lower than one might suspect. It is the *average* heart rate of the activity that is important. Other activities, such as walking, golf, and volleyball require only light energy expenditure and must be continued for relatively long periods in order to provide a training benefit.

The individual will be wise to base his personal fitness program on activities that fit his particular life situation. Some activities may be impractical to him because of time, money, or other factors. It is obvious that handball, basketball, tennis, and so on, require other players and courts for enjoyment. The unavailability of swimming, especially in the winter months, may eliminate this activity from one's program. In addition, the time which one can exercise may make it difficult to participate in these and similar activities.

Running is an exercise that makes for easy participation, and, at the same time, yields maximum benefits in terms of cardiovascular health. It is also inexpensive and less time consuming than most other activities. There is always a park, some other open land, or a street near one's home that can be utilized for a running area. The many advantages of running make it the most widely choosen activity in fitness programs. It is the first choice activity for cardiovascular conditioning. Bicycling should be rated second. It also places demands on large muscles and may be as strenuous as one chooses to make it.

CHAPTER 7   References

Balke, B. (1963). "A Simple Field Test for the Assessment of Physical Fitness." *Civil Aeromedical Research Institute Report* 63–6.

Banister, E. W., and Brown, S. R. (1968). "The Relative Energy Requirements of Physical Activity." *In Exercise Physiology* (H. B. Falls, ed.), pp. 268–322. Academic Press, New York.

Cooper, K. H. (1968a). *Aerobics*. Evans, New York.

Cooper, K. H. (1968b). "A Means of Assessing Maximal Oxygen Intake." *Journal of the American Medical Association* **203**:201–204.

Falls, H. B. (1969). "The Relative Energy Requirements of Various Physical Activities in Relation to Physiological Strain." *Journal of South Carolina Medical Association* **65** (13, Supplement I): 8–11.

Jackson, G. R. (1967). "The Effect of Training at Three Different Heart Rate Levels upon Cardiovascular Fitness." Unpublished master's thesis. Temple University, Philadelphia, Pennsylvania.

Karvonen, M. J. (1959). "Problems of Training the Cardiovascular System." *Ergonomics* **2**:207–215.

Karvonen, M. J., Kentala, E., and Mustala, O. (1957). "The Effects of Training on Heart Rate." *Annales Medicinae Experimentalis et Biologiae Fenniae (Helsinki)* **35**:307–315.

Passmore, R., and Durnin, J. V. G. A. (1955). "Human Energy Expenditure." *Physiological Reviews* **35**:801–835.

EIGHT / Nutrition, Weight Control, and Exercise

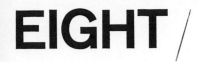

EIGHT /

There are an astonishing number of fads and falla-cies concerning the effect of diet and nutrition on physical performance and weight control. Nutritional practices based on hearsay and habit are often the rule rather than the exception. However, there is abundant information with which misconceptions may be dispelled.

I. FUNCTIONS OF FOOD

To properly nourish the body, foods must contain substances that function in one or more of three ways:

(1) furnish body fuel, substances whose oxidation in the body sets free energy needed for its activ-ities;
(2) provide materials for the building or mainte-nance of body tissues;
(3) supply substances that act to regulate body processes (Bogert, 1960).

An individual food may perform one of the above functions or all three. The diet as a whole *must* provide foods serving all three functions in order that good health may be maintained. A food that provides one or more of the functions is called a *nutrient*. Six classes of nutrients are necessary to the body. They are carbohydrates, fats, proteins, vitamins, mineral elements, and water. Since they are necessary to normal body functioning, they are called *essential nutrients*.

Body fuel is provided by carbohydrates, fats, and proteins. These substances are organic and are combustible. Fats, proteins, mineral elements, and water are essential in body composition and are, therefore, necessary for building and maintenance within the body tissues.

Mineral elements and vitamins regulate body functions by promoting oxidative processes, vitality of tissues, and normal functioning of nerves and muscles. In addition to being an important part of body structure, water serves as an important regulator by holding substances in solution in the digestive juices, blood, and tissues. It also aids in regulation of body temperature, circulation, and excretion.

It is often difficult to remember which foods must be included in the daily diet. As a helpful aid the U.S. Department of Agriculture has grouped foods into four main categories—Milk Group, Meat Group, Vegetables and Fruit, Breads and Cereals (United States Department of Agriculture, 1957). The following check list is provided to aid in food selection from these groups:

Milk Group—Two or more eight-ounce servings daily.

Children and teenagers need at least a quart. Ice cream and cheese may supply part of the needed amount. This group furnishes riboflavin (Vitamin B_2), Vitamin A, Vitamin D, and necessary proteins.

Meat Group—Two or more three-ounce servings daily.

This group includes meat, fish, cheese, legumes, eggs, nuts, and poultry. These foods are a prime source of needed protein, important vitamins, and iron.

Vegetable—Fruit Group—Four or five servings daily.

Green and yellow vegetables, one of them raw, should be included. Tomato juice or citrus fruit or juice should be provided daily. These are important suppliers of Vitamin C. Fruits and vegetables also supply Vitamin A and important minerals.

Bread—Cereals Group—Four to five servings daily.

Both bread and cereals should be used in the course of a week. This group is an excellent source of the B group of vitamins and Vitamin K.

If the indicated servings do not provide enough Calories for needed energy, additional amounts may be eaten from any of the four groups.

II. FOOD AS FUEL

To maintain life and perform work the body must have energy. In a sense it is an energy transforming machine. The source for all the energy transformations which occur within the body is ingested food. The basic unit of measurement for this energy is the kilocalorie (Calorie). The number of kilocalories needed by the body varies widely among individuals.

Virtually all the kilocalories of energy utilized by the body are supplied by four foods—carbohydrate, protein, fats, and ethanol (alcohol) (One should note that alcohol is not an essential food since it can do nothing more than supply kilocalories to the body). Carbohydrate is the prime source of body energy because it is more efficient in oxidation than the others. For each liter of oxygen consumed in oxidation of carbohydrate, 5.05 kilocalories of energy are produced. Oxidation of ethanol produces 4.86 kilocalories, while oxidation of fat and protein produce only 4.74 and 4.46 kilocalories per liter, respectively. Therefore, the body's energy needs should be met primarily through including foods rich in carbohydrate in the diet. Included in this category are granulated sugar, dry cereals, cookies, candy, cake, crackers, jams and jellies, dried fruits, legumes, white bread, potatoes, rice, spaghetti, and macaroni.

Fats are a secondary source of energy that is utilized if the carbohydrate supply is too low to meet the body's basic energy needs. This fact is used to good advantage in simple reducing diets by cutting down on the intake of both carbohydrate and fats. This causes the body to draw upon stored fat for oxidation thereby reducing the size of these deposits.

Protein is used for oxidation if both carbohydrate and fat supplies are inadequate, but this is rarely seen except in cases of severe nutritional inadequacies or in pathological conditions.

It is relatively easy to calculate the caloric value of one's diet since the number of kilocalories yielded by various foods has been scientifically determined and placed in tables such as Table 8.1. One need only calculate the amount of each food in the diet. With some practice one can become fairly accurate in these estimates.

Caloric values, such as those in Table 8.1, are calculated by burning food in an instrument known as a *bomb calorimeter*. It consists of a sealed container filled with pure oxygen to insure complete combustion. A known amount of food to be tested is placed in the chamber and ignited electrically. By measuring the heat released upon oxidation and dividing by the amount of food, the caloric value in kilocalories per gram can be calculated since one kilocalorie is the amount of heat necessary to raise the temperature of one kilogram of water one degree centigrade.

III. BODY ENERGY NEEDS

For determining all energy requirements of the body, a definite standard known as the basal metabolism is used. This may be defined as the minimum energy requirement, expressed in kilocalories, for each square meter of body surface area while the subject is awake but inactive. The measurement is usually taken before the subject rises from bed and before eating after a full night's sleep. Under these conditions, the basal metabolism of the body measures only the functional expenditure of energy necessary to maintain the body's internal processes such as heart beat, respiration, nervous system activity, and muscle tone. Under such conditions it has been found that the individual expends about 39.7 kilo-

Table 8.1
100-Kilocalorie Portions of Some Common Foods

Almonds	12
Apples	2
Apple sauce	⅜ cup
Asparagus	20 stalks
Bacon, fried	5 small slices
Bananas	1 large
Beans, baked	⅓ cup
Beans, string	2 cups
Beef, creamed dried	⅓ cup
Beef, roast	4 inches × 2 inches × ¼ inch serving
Beer	7 ounces
Blackberries	½ cup
Bread, white	1 thick slice
Butter	1 tablespoon
Cabbage	5 cups
Cake	1 thick slice, as of bread
Candy	1 ounce
Cantaloupe	1
Celery	1 bunch
Cheese	1 ounce
Cherries	1 cup fresh
Chocolates	1 medium
Cocktail, dry (sweet is more)	4 ounces
Cola drink	8 ounces
Corn, canned	⅓ cup
Cornflakes	1½ cups
Corn on cob	2 small ears
Cream	¼ cup
Cream of wheat, cooked	¾ cup
Cucumbers	3 medium
Dates	7
Egg, raw or cooked	1 large
Frankfurter	1 3½-inches long
Grape nuts	3 tablespoons
Grapes, Concord	1 large bunch
Haddock	large serving
Ham, roast	medium serving
Hickory nuts	15
Honey	1 tablespoon
Lemons	1 cup juice
Lettuce	2 large heads
Milk	⅝ glass (1 quart = 640 kilocalories)

Table 8.1 (continued)
100-Kilocalorie Portions of Some Common Foods

Oatmeal, cooked	1 cup
Orange	1 very large
Oysters	12 small
Peaches	3
Peanuts	10–12 double
Pears, canned	2 halves with juice
Peas	¾ cup
Pie	1½-inch sector of a 9-inch diameter pie
Potatoes, boiled	1 large
Potatoes, mashed	½ cup
Raisins	¼ cup
Roll	1
Salmon	medium serving
Sardines	3–6
Shredded wheat	1 biscuit
Spinach	2½ cups
Steak, hamburger	1 medium cake
Steak, tenderloin	2 inches × 1 inch × 1 inch serving
Tomatoes, canned	1¾ cup
Tomatoes, stuffed	1
Veal roast	medium serving
Waffles	½
Walnuts	10

calories of energy per hour for each square meter of body surface area. Normally, the individual should not deviate more than 10 percent from this standard (Hickman, 1968).

Tables presenting such basal data are usually based on the "standard or reference man," who is 5 feet 7 inches tall and weighs 154 pounds or 70 kilograms. He thus has a body surface area of 1.80 square meters and requires about 70 kilocalories per hour (1.80 × 39.7) for basal metabolic needs. If one varies much in size from the "standard man" he will need to compute his own body surface area before he can make an accurate estimate of his basal metabolic energy needs. This can be accomplished by utilizing the body surface area calculations of Figure 8.1. A man six feet tall and weighing 180 pounds, for example, would have a body surface area of 2.04 square meters and corresponding basal

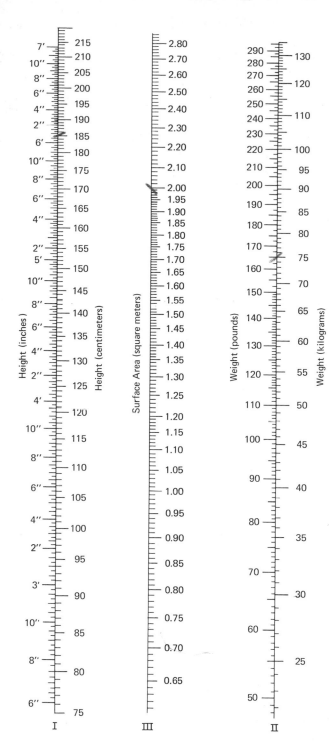

FIGURE 8.1   Dubois Body Surface Chart (As prepared by Boothby and Sandiford of the Mayo Clinic). To find the body surface area of a subject, locate the height in inches (or centimeters) on Scale I and the weight in pounds (or kilograms) on Scale III and place a straight edge (ruler) between these two points. The straight edge will intersect Scale II at the subject's surface area (Reproduced from "Clinical Spirometry" through courtesy of Warren E. Collins, Braintree, Massachusetts).

metabolic energy need of about 81 kilocalories per hour (39.7 × 2.04).

Daily calorie needs obviously far exceed these basal requirements. To determine total calorie needs the "active" metabolic requirements must be assessed as well. The following example should provide the background for computation of total caloric needs. Our subject above needed 81 kilocalories per hour for basal metabolism. This is a total of 1944 for the day (24 × 81). Table 8.2 presents kilocalorie expenditures of various activities per kilogram of body weight. This table can be used to complete our estimates. Let us suppose our subject is a fairly

Table 8.2
Kilocalories per Hour Expended in Various Activities*

Activity	Kilocalories per hour per kilogram body weight†
Sitting	0.3
Standing	0.5
Playing pool	0.6
Singing	0.7
Dressing	0.8
Driving a car	0.9
Typing	1.0
Piano playing	1.4
House work	1.6
Walking (3 miles per hour)	2.0
Volleyball	2.1
Carpentry	2.4
Golf	3.0
Ping pong	3.1
Dancing	3.8
Tennis	5.0
Climbing upstairs	5.8
Basketball	6.0
Swimming (recreational)	6.0
Jogging (5 miles per hour)	7.0
Bicycling (moderate speed)	8.4
Handball	9.3
Swim (crawl)	11.0
Running (8–10 miles per hour)	11.9
Sprinting	18.7

* Based on data presented by Passmore and Durnin (1955) and Banister and Brown (1968).

† These values do not include basal metabolic needs.

active college student who spent the day as follows: 8 hours sleep, 10 hours sitting in class, studying, eating, talking, etc., 1 hour walking, ½ hour driving a car, 1 hour playing basketball, 1 hour playing ping pong, 1 hour at a dance, 15 minutes climbing stairs, and 15 minutes running at 5 miles per hour in a physical education class. Using Table 8.2 we would calculate the energy expenditures below. Ten percent of this value must be added to cover the energy cost of food digestion. His total caloric expenditure would thus be 4058. (*Note:* 1 hour of walking requires two thirds as much energy as sitting for 10 hours.)

1944	basal metabolism
243	$(10 \times 0.3 \times 81)$ sitting
162	$(1 \times 2 \times 81)$ walking
36	$(½ \times 0.9 \times 81)$ driving
486	$(1 \times 6.0 \times 81)$ basketball
251	$(1 \times 3.1 \times 81)$ ping pong
308	$(1 \times 3.8 \times 81)$ dancing
117	$(¼ \times 5.8 \times 81)$ stairs
142	$(¼ \times 7 \times 81)$ running
3689	
369	digestion of food
4058	Total

IV KILOCALORIE BALANCE

It is obvious that the objective, under normal conditions, is to achieve a balance between the expenditure of kilocalories as in the example above and the intake of kilocalories from food. If an imbalance does exist it will result in either a loss or possibly a gain in weight. If more kilocalories than needed for energy expenditure are consumed, a weight gain usually results. The reverse is always true. When the diet supplies less than is needed, the energy requirement must come from sources stored in the body. In the case of an oversupply, our body usually stores the extra energy in the form of fat deposits. Some fortunate people need not worry about overeating, at least while they are young. If an undersupply exists, the body oxidizes first, stored fat deposits and secondly, in the case of severe nutritional deficiencies, protein. One can determine whether his kilocalorie equation balances by utilization of Tables 8.1 and 8.2. Making these calculations for one day is not adequate since either food intake, energy expenditure, or both may vary quite drastically from the average on any single day. To get a truer picture one should compute an average based on a two to three week period. The following sections will explain how the results of this calculation can be utilized in setting up and carrying out a weight control program.

V. WEIGHT CONTROL

A. Overweight and Obesity

In an inactive, sedentary society overweight and obesity are serious health problems. Although weight control is not a problem for everyone, it concerns a major portion of the adult population. To those beset with overweight or underweight difficulties, control of weight is a time, energy, and too often, money consuming problem. Although weight control theories and practices are relatively simple, there is an alarming amount of confusion. Millions of dollars are spent annually on weight reduction nostrums and schemes advertised as "easy, quick, pleasant, and permanent." The abundance of remedies is rivaled only by the number of unsatisfied participants. Sound knowledge used correctly is the best method of controlling body weight.

Overweight and obesity may be due to emotional stress in which the individual gains satisfaction from eating, a glandular condition, overeating, or lack of exercise. The preceding conditions may be present singly or in combination. The diet is most frequently involved, and treatment is usually successful when dietary corrections are made. In situations where the obesity is due to something other than overeating and/or lack of exercise, it is best to obtain medical advice. In any event, especially important is the rate and manner in which a person reduces his weight. It should be lost gradually, and care should be taken to insure that all essential nutrients are included in adequate amounts in any reducing diet.

1. OBESITY DEFINED

A distinction may be made between what is considered overweight and obesity. Overweight means being of above average weight, while being obese means the deposit of excessive body fat. One who is overweight is not necessarily obese. It may simply mean that he has a body weight somewhat greater than average for his age and height. However, one who exceeds 20 percent over average weight is generally considered obese. We are primarily concerned with obesity since it poses several threats to health.

2. HAZARDS OF OBESITY

Through extensive research on the problem of obesity, a number of specific hazards to general health and well-being have been identified. These hazards include:

(1) greater risk of developing and suffering from hypertension, atherosclerosis, diabetes, gall bladder disease, degenerative arthritis, and kidney disease (Armstrong et al., 1951; Marks, 1957);
(2) adverse postural changes;
(3) delayed puberty in children;
(4) decreased endurance (Dempsey, 1964);
(5) increased mortality rates (Death rates among obese men average 50 percent higher than expectancies) (Armstrong et al., 1951).

It has already been stated that a desirable objective for the person of normal body weight is a balance of kilocalorie intake and expenditure. If this balance is not achieved, either underweight or obesity may be the end result. In our society obesity develops far more often than underweight. In fact, it is the most common uncorrected physical defect of Americans. By adulthood at least 25 percent of the population is in various stages of obesity, some of it acute. This "creeping obesity" can be observed merely by a critical look at college students on any campus.

3. DETERMINING YOUR OBESITY STATUS

It is relatively easy for one to determine if he is overweight or obese. He may start by consulting a table of average weights such as that published by the Metropolitan Life Insurance Company (Table 8.3). If he is above the listed weights for his height and body frame, it does not necessarily mean he is obese. It may simply mean he is more heavily muscled and of heavier bone structure than the average man of his physical proportions.

Conversely, even if he is within the average ranges he may still be obese. His ratio of fat to total weight may be excessively high. This is actually the key to obesity—the amount of fat in relation to the total weight of the body. Obviously, the lower the fat weight of the body in relation to total pounds the less one is likely to be obese. There are some sophisticated tests of obesity in which the "lean body mass" is estimated through immersing the total body in water and measuring the amount of water displaced. Other techniques involve measuring the thickness of "fat folds" at various points on the body, but most people can simply look at themselves and determine if they carry excessive fat.

B. Weight Control through Exercise

The means of losing weight are relatively simple. Either one must increase his kilocalorie expenditure through activity or reduce intake by diet. If this is done, the stored fat will be utilized for body fuel and literally be "burned off." A combination of reduced intake and increased expenditure is probably best. Increased exercise is the most desirable alternative because one can reduce his body weight and at the same time build up increased physical fitness. Another advantage of exercise in achieving a kilocalorie deficit is advocated by nutrition experts who have observed that individuals who exercise regularly tend to regulate their kilocalorie intake according to their individual need (Mayer, 1968). This means that one need not necessarily go on a reducing diet.

Table 8.2 shows kilocalorie expenditures for various physical activities. It can be used as a guide in determining how much extra daily activity one needs on a reducing program. Running and walking can be used to good advantage because it is quite easy to determine exactly how many kilocalories are ex-

Table 8.3
Average Weights for Different Body Types*

Height		Small	Medium	Large
Feet	Inches	Frame	Frame	Frame
5	2	112–120	118–129	126–141
5	3	115–123	121–133	129–144
5	4	118–126	124–136	132–148
5	5	121–129	127–139	135–152
5	6	124–133	130–143	138–156
5	7	128–137	134–147	142–161
5	8	132–141	138–152	147–166
5	9	136–145	142–156	151–170
5	10	140–150	146–160	155–174
5	11	144–154	150–165	159–179
6	0	148–158	154–170	164–184
6	1	152–162	158–175	168–189
6	2	156–167	162–180	173–194
6	3	160–171	167–185	178–199
6	4	164–175	172–190	182–204

* With shoes and ordinary clothing. (Courtesy Metropolitan Life Insurance Company—From Statistical Bulletin Volume 40, November–December, 1959.)

pended when one covers a certain distance. R. P. Margaria, a noted Italian physiologist, has demonstrated that, regardless of speed, one will expend one kilocalorie per kilogram body weight for each 1000 meters he covers walking or running (Margaria et al., 1963). In Table 8.4 kilocalorie expenditures have been worked out for various body weights and distances. By utilization of this table one can get a very close estimate of the number of kilocalories he expends when walking or running. For example, in order for a 180 pound man to nullify the kilocalorie effect of a 12 ounce beer (180 kilocalories), he needs to run or walk approximately 1½ miles. Think

Table 8.4
Kilocalories Expended in Walking and/or
Running Various Distances for Different Body Weights

Body weight	Miles			
	1	1½	2	2½
140	103	154	205	257
160	117	176	235	293
180	132	199	265	330
200	146	221	295	332
220	160	243	325	402
240	174	265	355	438

how far he would need to run to nullify a six-pack.

A deficit of 3500 kilocalories is required in order to remove a pound of stored fat. This is equivalent to a daily kilocalorie deficit of 500 if one wishes to lose one pound per week. Medical authorities recommend that not more than about two pounds per week be lost. Therefore, one needs a daily kilocalorie deficit of no more than 1000. Two pounds per week is considerable weight loss when one considers this would total 104 pounds if carried on for a year.

C. Body Composition

1. IMPORTANCE OF FAT-FREE BODY WEIGHT

It has been pointed out that high percentages of fat in relation to total body weight are detrimental and lead to obesity. The lower the fat content of the body, the higher the so-called "fat-free" body weight. Research has shown that the relative degree of fat-free body weight is not only important from a health standpoint, but it is an important factor contributing to higher levels of human physical performance in activities where the body weight must be moved (Leedy et al., 1965). Also, high percentages of body fat lessen the relative ability to supply oxygen to the body tissues thus cutting down on one's cardiovascular endurance (Falls et al., 1965).

Excess body fat in a certain area of the body acts in much the same manner as would an equal weight object strapped around that part of the anatomy (for example, it places an unnecessary extra load on the physiological functions of the body).

2. AGE AND EXERCISE EFFECTS

Percentage of total body weight that is fat-free shows a steady decline with increasing age after 20 years among the male population. This is a reflection of increasing accumulations of body fat generally due to more sedentary living habits. Exercise has been shown to be effective in offsetting and/or delaying this trend. Individuals who exercise regularly are able to maintain their fat-free weight in later years closer to that of their young adulthood than are those who do not (Consolazio et al., 1963; Ismail, 1968). This is an important consideration in view of the high percentage of heart disease due to obesity in our society.

Changes in body composition are very important also from a motivational standpoint in exercise programs. A person who is obese may begin an exercise program expecting to lose weight and he may not. In fact, he may gain weight. This often occurs in individuals who are low in strength and muscular development. Body fat is lost, but it is replaced by muscle tissue. If weight loss is the chief motivation for the exercise, then the individual may be disappointed with the results. He should keep in mind that it is the body composition—the amount of fat-free weight—that is important. Although he has lost no weight, he will probably have lost inches around the waist and elsewhere and will have a trimmer appearance.

3. SPOT REDUCING

Many individuals attempt to effect specific weight reduction by concentrating on the body spots which have greatest fat accumulation. Mechanical vibrators, belt massagers, and similar devices are predicated on this assumption, and large profits are obtained yearly from a gullible public.

A summary of the available research indicates that spot reducing using *specific local exercises* "may be effective but probably no more so than general 'nonspot' exercise of equal intensity and duration" (Johnson et al., 1966; Carns et al., 1960). Most of the positive results are probably attributable to development of better muscle tone in the involved areas.

Scientific evidence favoring the use of mechanical vibrating devices is lacking, but research studies have been conducted that indicate they are ineffective. One study showed that the energy expenditure involved in walking up one flight of stairs was equivalent to that of 45 minutes in a mechanical vibrator (Karpovich, 1960). Another found that it would take 94 hours of vibration to lose a pound of fat (Steinhaus, 1963). In view of these findings, an individual would be foolish to make use of these devices.

VI. NUTRITION AND PHYSICAL PERFORMANCE

There are many misconceptions among coaches, trainers, and athletes, as well as the general public about the role of various foodstuffs in relation to physical performance. Many feel there are "super-foods" that should be eaten regularly. Others feel that what is eaten in a "pre-event" meal is highly significant. Based on the available scientific research, the following guidelines seem reasonable:

(1) If the individual is following a well-balanced diet based on the United States Department of Agriculture recommendations he is not likely to receive benefit from adding so-called "superfoods" to the diet, for instance, dextrose tablets, wheat germ, and so on.

(2) Little significance can be attached to the "pre-event" meal *if* (a) the diet is already balanced, (b) the individual eats foods that he normally eats, (c) the meal is not large, (d) it is not taken immediately prior to exercise, (e) it is not excessive in protein intake if the event is an endurance activity (Guild, 1960).

(3) There is no such thing as the "athletic diet." The diet of the athlete must contain all the essential nutrients just as that of the nonathlete. In addition, his food intake must be greater to take care of the increased caloric expenditure of exercise. To this end extra quantities of carbohydrate foods are normally included in the diet (Ahlborg et al., 1967).

(4) Care should be taken not to allow too much time to elapse between the time the last meal is taken and exercise begins. This time interval, especially if the exercise is to be prolonged, probably should be no more than four hours. Beyond this point one runs the risk of allowing the blood sugar to drop below normal resting levels. If this situation occurs, energy supplies are not as readily available to the individual. Also, the liver stores about 1000 Calories which is sufficient to sustain about one hour of vigorous activity. If too much time elapses before activity this energy resource is depleted.

CHAPTER 8   References

Ahlborg, B., Bergstrom, J., Brohult, J., Ekelund, L., Hultman, E., and Maschio, G. (1967). "Human Muscle Glycogen Content and Capacity for Prolonged Exercise after Different Diets." *Försvarsmedicin* **3**:85–100.

Armstrong, D. B., Dublin, L. I., Wheatley, G. M., and Marks, H. H. (1951). "Obesity and Its Relation to Health and Disease." *Journal of the American Medical Association* **147**:1007–1014.

Banister, E. W., and Brown, S. R. (1968). "The Relative Energy Requirements of Physical Activity." *In Exercise Physiology* (H. B. Falls, ed.), pp. 268–322. Academic Press, New York.

Bogert, L. J. (1960). *Nutrition and Physical Fitness.* Saunders, Philadelphia, Pennsylvania.

Carns, M. L., Schade M. L., Liba, M. R., Hellebrandt, F. A., and Harris, C. W. (1960). "Segmental Volume Reduction by Localized versus Generalized Exercise." *Human Biology* **32**:370–376.

Consolazio, C. F., Johnson, R. E., and Pecora, L. J. (1963). *Physiological Measurements of Metabolic Functions in Man.* McGraw-Hill, New York.

Dempsey, J. A. (1964). "Relationship between Obesity and Treadmill Performance in Sedentary and Active Young Men." *Research Quarterly of the American Association for Health, Physical Education and Recreation* **35**:288–297.

Falls, H. B., Ismail, A. H., MacLeod, D. F., Wiebers, J. E., Christian, J. E., and Kessler, M. V. (1965). "Development of Physical Fitness Test Batteries by Factor Analysis Techniques." *Journal of Sports Medicine and Physical Fitness* **5**:185–197.

Guild, W. (1960). "Pre-event Nutrition, with Some Implications for Endurance Athletes." *In Exercise and Fitness*, pp. 135–137. Athletic Institute, Chicago, Illinois.

Hickman, C. P. (1968). *Health for College Students.* Prentice-Hall, Englewood Cliffs, New Jersey.

Ismail, A. H. (1968). "Body Composition and Relationships to Physical Activity." *In Exercise Physiology* (H. B. Falls, ed.), pp. 387–392. Academic Press, New York.

Johnson, P. B., Updyke, W. F., Stolberg, D. C., and Schaefer, M. (1966). *Physical Education: A Problem-Solving Approach to Health and Fitness.* Holt, New York.

Karpovich, P. V. (1960). "Ergogenic Aids in Athletics." *In Exercise and Fitness*, pp. 82–90. Athletic Institute, Chicago, Illinois.

Leedy, H. E., Ismail, A. H., Kessler, M. V., and Christian, J. E. (1965). "Relationships between Physical Performance Items and Body Composition." *Research Quarterly of the American Association for Health, Physical Education and Recreation* **36**:158–163.

Margaria, R., Cerretelli, P., Aghemo, P., and Sassi, G. (1963). "Energy Cost of Running." *Journal of Applied Physiology* **18**:367–370.

Marks, H. H. (1957). "Relationship of Body Weight to Mortality and Morbidity." *Metabolism, Clinical and Experimental* **6**:417–424.

Mayer, J. (1968). *Overweight: Causes, Cost, and Control.* Prentice-Hall, Englewood Cliffs, New Jersey.

Passmore, R., and Durnin, J. V. G. A. (1955). "Human Energy Expenditure." *Physiological Reviews* **35**:801–835.

Steinhaus, A. H. (1963). *Toward an Understanding of Health and Physical Education.* W. C. Brown, Dubuque, Iowa.

United States Department of Agriculture (1957). "Essentials of an Adequate Diet, Home Economics Research Report No. 3." United States Department of Agriculture.

APPENDIXES/

APPENDIX A
Muscles of the Body—
front view.
  (1) Sternocleido-
mastoideus
  (2) Trapezius
  (3) Deltoid
  (4) Pectoralis major
  (5) Serratus anterior
  (6) Biceps brachii
  (7) External oblique
  (8) Rectus abdominis
  (9) Vastus lateralis
 (10) Rectus femoris
 (11) Vastus medialis
 (12) Gastrocnemius
 (13) Soleus

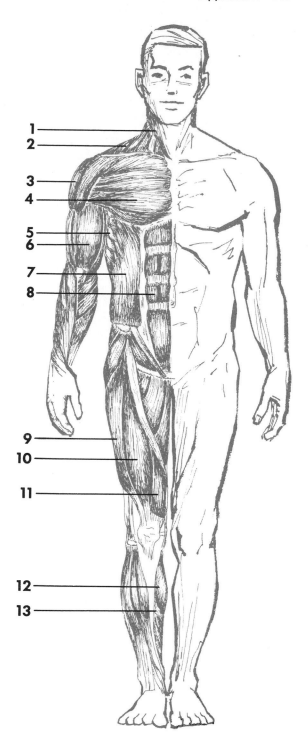

APPENDIX B
Muscles of the Body—
back view.
 (1) Trapezius
 (2) Deltoid
 (3) Teres major
 (4) Triceps brachii
 (5) Latissimus dorsi
 (6) Gluteus maximus
 (7) Biceps femoris
 (8) Semitendinosus
 (9) Semimembranosus
(10) Gastrocnemius
(11) Soleus

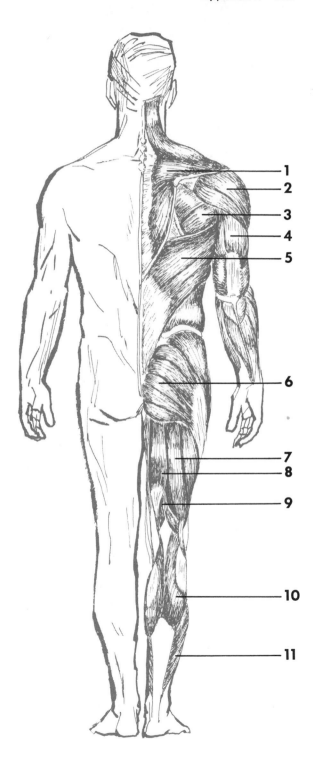